GETTING THE WORD OUT

A Practical Guide to AIDS Materials Development

▲▲▲▲▲▲

Edited by Ana Consuelo Matiella

PRODUCED FOR THE CALIFORNIA AIDS CLEARINGHOUSE, A PROJECT OF
ETR ASSOCIATES, WITH FUNDS FROM THE CALIFORNIA OFFICE OF AIDS
SANTA CRUZ, CALIFORNIA ▲ 1990

© 1990 by Network Publications, a division of ETR
Associates. Produced for the California AIDS
Clearinghouse, a project of ETR Associates, with
funds from the California Office of AIDS. Published
by Network Publications, P.O. Box 1830, Santa Cruz,
CA 95061-1830.
Printed in the United States of America
Cover and text design: Lance Sprague

10 9 8 7 6 5 4 3 2

Table of Contents

Appendixes

Preface

Getting the Word Out provides health educators with a practical guide for developing effective AIDS education materials. The underlying message within the book, however, is deeper. More than merely a materials development guide, this book also provides insights and recommendations on how to make educational materials culturally sensitive and relevant to the diverse communities they are intended to reach.

We believe that this book can be a rich resource, not only for AIDS educators, but for all health educators who can stand to learn and grow from the valuable if painful lessons that AIDS continues to teach us.

The book offers a collection of chapters on the specifics of the materials development process; it also translates some intangible cultural nuances into practical information that is vital to consider as one goes through this challenging process.

In these pages we have provided a variety of points of view as well as diverse professional and cultural perspectives. This diverse representation is just one feature that adds to the richness and depth of the book.

Getting the Word Out is intended to be a reflection of the philosophy that educational materials need to be responsive to the specific needs of the populations being served, and that the more specifically targeted materials are, the better they are at achieving their educational objectives.

Because we espouse this philosophy, we believe that local communities are best equipped to design and develop materials that will meet their own unique needs. We see our role as health educators (and materials developers) as facilitators of a process, and we believe that this process is most successful when it is a participatory community effort. We hope this book helps you enhance this effort.

Ana Consuelo Matiella, MA
Editor

Acknowledgments

Special thanks to the following people who participated in the conceptualization, critique and final review of the manuscript:

The California AIDS Clearinghouse (CAC) Advisory Board

Priscilla Alexander
California Prostitute Education
Project (CAL-PEP)
San Francisco, California

Elena Alvarado
Avance Human Services
Los Angeles, California

José Aponte
San Juan Capistrano Regional
Library
San Juan Capistrano, California

Paul Causey
UCSF AIDS Health Project
San Francisco, California

Lianne B. Chong
L. Chong Designs Associates
San Francisco, California

James W. Dilley
UCSF AIDS Health Project
San Francisco, California

Peggy Falk
Humboldt/Del Norte Counties
Public Health Department
Eureka, California

Estella Garcia
Instituto Familiar de la Raza
San Francisco, California

Diane Gray
Asian AIDS Project
San Francisco, California

Craig Lasha
Mid-City Consortium to
Combat AIDS
San Francisco, California

Milton Lee
King Drew Medical Center
Los Angeles, California

Tom Lidot
San Diego American Indian
Health Center
San Diego, California

Chente Matus
Mid-City Consortium to
Combat AIDS
San Francisco, California

John Mortimer
AIDS Project Los Angeles
Los Angeles, California

Ricardo Perugorría
Community Health Centers of
Kern County
Bakersfield, California

Russell Toth
California AIDS Information
Network (CAIN)
Hollywood, California

Sala Udin
Multicultural AIDS Resource
Center
San Francisco, California

Dean Yabuki
East Bay Asian AIDS
Coordinating Committee
Oakland, California

Getting the Word Out Reviewers

José Aponte
San Juan Capistrano Regional
Library
San Juan Capistrano, California

Alma Berrow
City of Berkeley
Office of Planning, Education
and Promotion
Berkeley, California

Paul Causey
AIDS Health Project
San Francisco, California

Peggy Falk
Humboldt County Health
Department
Eureka, California

Ruth Lopez
Salud Para La Gente, Inc.
Watsonville, California

Connie Madden
AIDS Program Development
Associate
San Francisco, California

Linda Okahara and Kevin
Fong
Asian Health Services
Oakland, California

Ricardo Perugorría
Community Health Centers of
Kern County
Bakersfield, California

Sam Radelfinger
Health Education Department
San Jose State University
San Jose, California

Richard Rios
Madera Public Health
Department
Madera, California

Dean Yabuki
East Bay Asian AIDS
Coordinating Committee
Oakland, California

Introduction

Getting the Word Out is a collection of chapters written by community AIDS educators who have specialized knowledge and skill in developing educational materials in multi-ethnic communities. The overall goal of this book is to give tangible, specific and useful information to health professionals on how to develop effective AIDS education materials. Equally important is the information that will help enhance the cultural sensitivity and relevance of materials.

This book is about materials development, and as such, has its limitations. Materials development is but one aspect of a well-planned and effective AIDS education program. Because the focus of this book is on materials development, it is important to keep in mind that printed materials are meant to be support materials. They are not meant to be a substitute for the personal interaction and benefit derived from face-to-face communication.

How to Use This Book

We have presented the chapters in what seemed to be the most appropriate order—to reflect the process of materials development—beginning with chapters on needs assessment and research. However, we encourage you to read the book in the order that best suits your needs, revisiting the most relevant chapters according to the particular tasks that you and your community are working on at the present time.

Each chapter is meant to stand alone. As you read, you may find that points of information are repeated across some of the chapters. In each chapter, we chose to leave the message intact—allowing the uniqueness of the different perspectives and approaches to shine through.

What Is in This Book

The first three chapters of the book are about assessing the needs of the community through various methods. Chapter 1, "Laying the Groundwork," emphasizes the importance of assessing community needs for effective program planning. Knowing your community, identifying target groups and behaviors at risk, and researching demographics and rates of infection are some of the issues covered here. The author also provides a list of pertinent questions to ask before embarking on a community needs assessment.

"Using Evaluation to Develop Responsive Materials" details how to use evaluation to shape the development of the materials. This chapter highlights a 6-step framework that focuses on process. "Using Focus Group Interviews to Design Materials" discusses the purpose and appropriate use of focus group interviews and provides step-by-step guidelines on how to organize, facilitate and interpret their results.

In Chapter 4, "Creating Culturally Sensitive Materials," the author addresses this delicate process with a checklist of questions as criteria for developing effective and culturally sensitive educational materials. The chapter also provides an indepth look at three diverse communities and how each dealt with this challenge.

In the next nine chapters, a number of experts in the field devote their attention to the specifics of the actual development process. "Developing Low-Literacy Materials" provides how-to information on developing materials for low-literacy readers. The author suggests ways to simplify text and ideas, and recommends the use of pictures and illustrations to convey messages.

"Adapting and Translating Materials" discusses the appropriate and inappropriate use of translations and adaptations, identifies key developmental steps to keep in mind, and offer some hints on how to hire a developer to do the work.

"Singing Your Own Song" provides an insightful analysis on the cross-cultural implications of doing adaptations, and makes some concrete suggestions on how to improve materials from an intercultural perspective. "Telling a Tale" is a concrete account of how to use traditional communication channels to "get the word out."

With the recent surge of photoliterature and comic books as health education tools, "Producing Comic Books and Photonovels" adds another timely and useful dimension to the book. This brief overview outlines the developmental steps of a photonovel *(fotonovela)* project. "Developing Relevant Materials on a Low Budget" is rich with suggestions and observations gained from the author's experience. This chapter also addresses issues of cultural relevance and sensitivity.

The mystery of the production process is solved in

"Understanding the Production Process." The author provides a no-nonsense look at what goes into creating a finished product and provides realistic suggestions on how to get good quality and cost-effective work with a minimum of professional stress.

The last two chapters of *Getting the Word Out* focus on two very important aspects of our work: outreach and dissemination, and evaluating materials.

The author of "Planning Outreach and Dissemination Strategies," an outreach worker and health educator, outlines the most important characteristics of effective outreach. "Evaluating AIDS Education Materials" supplies the reader with a pragmatic look at the final evaluation process.

Appendixes

There are three case studies provided in the appendix section of the book. Appendix A, "Assessing the AIDS Education Needs of Black Gay and Bisexual Men," is a study based on behavior reported in a confidential survey in Baltimore, Maryland and Washington, D.C.

Appendix B is "Stopping AIDS is My Mission (SAMM)." This is a practical application of the work that Dr. Aisha Gilliam did in Chapter 2, "Using Evaluation to Develop Reponsive Materials."

Appendix C is an explanation of the Community Health Outreach Worker (CHOW) program and how it is used in street outreach. All appendixes are intended to provide tangible examples of going beyond the materials development process.

It is our hope that *Getting the Word Out* will be a resource that will prove useful and practical as you do your work. We are confident that we have taken another step toward the continued improvement of AIDS education.

1

Laying the Groundwork

Stephen B. Thomas, PhD

Introduction

The purpose of this chapter is to describe basic community needs assessment methods as the initial step in program planning and evaluation. Specifically, the goal is to increase the likelihood that community-based organizations (CBOs) will be able to demonstrate effectiveness in overcoming knowledge deficits, attitudinal barriers and risk behaviors for human immunodeficiency virus (HIV) infection in selected communities.

What are the specific AIDS education needs of your community? The correct answer to this question must emerge from knowledge about individuals, groups and institutions that make up your community. The correct answer must be based upon the means by which the AIDS virus is known to be transmitted. The correct answer must be based upon knowledge and insight about selected groups within your community that practice behaviors that increase the risk of HIV infection. The correct answer must be sensitive to the perceived needs and values of residents in the community.

The overrepresentation of ethnic populations among reported AIDS cases indicates a need for prevention strategies that specifically target ethnic communities as well as sub-groups within the ethnic communities. Ethnographically, within each "target community" there is a complex world of ever-changing meanings and behaviors. Effective prevention strategies aimed at changing behavior must take into account cultural and behavioral patterns, socioeconomic factors, social norms and a deeper understanding of language usage in the ethnic community.

To date, relatively few research efforts have targeted ethnic populations. Those which have include Holmberg (1987), Bausell (1986), DiClemente and Boyer (1987), and Strunin and Hingson (1987). These research projects have examined AIDS myths, fears, knowledge and attitudes of selected population groups.

Additionally, Thomas, Gilliam and Iwrey (1989) have reported that educational interventions designed to reduce high-risk behaviors have not focused on specific ethnic groups—and some that have reinforce the misconceptions already in place in the community.

The Nation of Islam, for example, has disseminated literature in the Black community purporting AIDS as a form of genocide, an attempt by White society to eliminate the Black race. More recently, findings by TRESP Associates, Thomas, Gilliam and Seltzer indicate a need to become aware of sub-cultural populations within ethnic communities to target accurate, acceptable, and culturally appropriate risk-reduction interventions.

This complex cultural web presents a formidable challenge for program planning and evaluation. Before we examine the steps needed to conduct a community needs assessment, it may be useful to provide an overview of the program evaluation process.

A Brief Overview of Program Evaluation

Accounting for Change

The essential purpose of evaluation, accounting for change, is often broken down into subcomponents. The first step in evaluation is taken to improve program planning and implementation so as to increase program effects or outcomes. These initial evaluations are called **formative evaluations** because they are designed to help form the program itself (see Figure 1.1).

The second step in evaluation (see Figure 1.2) is deciding whether a program should be continued, replicated, or selected from among two or more alternatives. Such evaluations are called **summative evaluations** because they are designed to help determine whether the

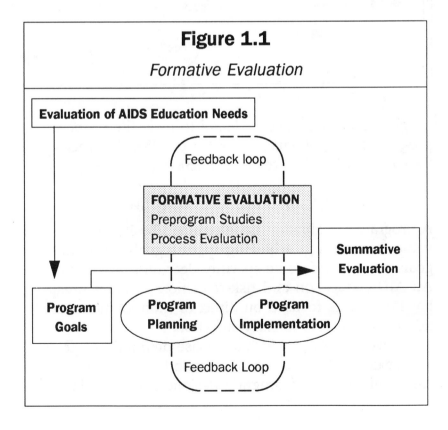

Figure 1.1

Formative Evaluation

Evaluation of AIDS Education Needs

Feedback loop

FORMATIVE EVALUATION
Preprogram Studies
Process Evaluation

Summative Evaluation

Program Goals

Program Planning

Program Implementation

Feedback Loop

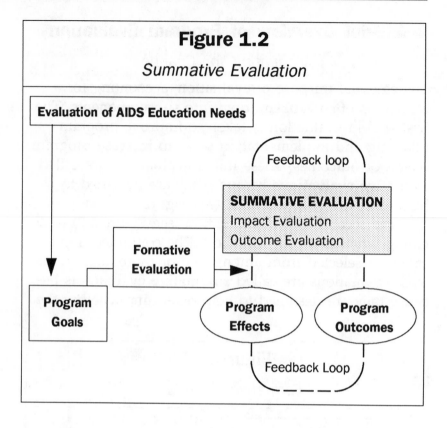

Figure 1.2

Summative Evaluation

program has succeeded or failed to meet the proposed program goals (Thomas, 1990; Fetro, 1989; Posavac, Carey, 1980; Rossie, Freeman, 1985).

Program Goals and Objectives

A program's evaluation is determined by its relative value or success in achieving specific goals. Program goals must therefore be specific, clear and measurable. An AIDS education and risk-reduction program must have objectives focused on direct or indirect modification of risk factors for HIV infection.

Dever (1980) provides a concise definition of goals and objectives. Confusion over these two terms may create time delays if program designers are unable to reach consensus. The following should help clarify the difference between them. Goals are general and abstract ways of stating desirable human health conditions. They may be expressed as quantifiable, timeless aspirations. Goals should also be technically and financially achievable and responsive to community ideals. Objectives, on the other hand, are specific and operational statements regarding the desired accomplishments of the AIDS education intervention. Objectives should express particular levels of expected achievements in health status by a specific year (Dever, 1980; Rossi, Freeman, 1985). For example:

Goal: Provide effective AIDS education and risk reduction programs to Black men at risk for HIV infection in Prince George's County Maryland.

Objective: By 1995, the availability of AIDS prevention programs and risk reduction methods (education, counseling, and medical services) to Black men should have sufficiently increased so as to reduce by 50 percent the HIV infection rate disparity between Black men and White men in Prince George's County Maryland.

Setting goals and specifying objectives require either assumptions or knowledge about the existing community conditions. The goal to reach Black men with effective AIDS prevention and risk-reduction methods assumes the importance of education, counseling and medical services in the reduction of risk factors for HIV infection. This goal is based on the assumption that there is room for improvement...that there is some significant discrepancy between the actual conditions and the desired outcome of implementing a program. Although a deficiency in existing conditions may be easy to recognize, a precise assessment using figures or statistics is usually required before realistic goals, objectives and program plans can be implemented (Rossi, et al., 1985).

How many goals and objectives should be included in AIDS risk-reduction programs? It is important to consider how much the community can accomplish. The AIDS risk-reduction program plan should include priority health status goals and objectives developed according to recommendations and resource requirements. Thus, in setting goal priorities, criteria such as the **extent of the problem, agency resources** and **feasibility of impacting** on the problem must be considered. The AIDS education program planner should be aware of the following considerations when establishing AIDS risk-reduction goals and objectives:

▲ Appropriate operational definitions of goals and objectives are related to the planning process.

▲ Quantitative goals and objectives (i.e., attainment levels) result from community and professional inputs as well as from data analysis.

▲ The number of goals and objectives must be appropriate for the problem, the feasibility of impacting on the problem, and the availability of agency resources.

▲ The kinds of goals and objectives are a reflection of the AIDS education program policies, national priorities, and needs assessment.

Many community-based organizations will need technical assistance to accomplish this fundamental task of establishing program goals and objectives. A comprehensive community needs assessment is the first step in the process.

The Need for Needs Assessment

We can define the needs assessment as the initial step in program planning. The assessment method must include a composite package of risk-reduction interventions that are most appropriate and cost-effective for the target population (Green and Lewis, 1986). The needs assessment thus helps lay the groundwork for program planning and evaluation. An evaluation of program effectiveness is only meaningful and useful if it follows an accurate assessment of needs.

The following four components represent the minimum outcome of the needs assessment process. The items listed below each component will vary by community but demonstrate the type of information to be gathered.

1   Characteristics and health status of the community
   • leading causes of illness and death
   • specific risk factors associated with leading causes of illness and death
   • incidence and prevalence of AIDS
   • incidence and prevalence of HIV infection
   • incidence and prevalence of risk factors for HIV infection

2   Characteristics of existing health care delivery systems in the community
   • availability of HIV testing and counseling
   • availability of primary medical care for persons with AIDS
   • availability of drug abuse treatment programs
   • availability and content of existing AIDS education programs

3   Which factors are most likely to be influenced by educational interventions
   • knowledge about AIDS and transmission of HIV

- attitudes and beliefs about AIDS and people with AIDS (PWAs)
- sexual behavior
- drug use behavior

4   Which AIDS risk-reduction services require priority
- treatment for persons living with AIDS
- HIV counseling and testing for persons at risk for HIV infection
- modification of high-risk sexual behavior
- modification of high-risk drug use behavior
- increased community awareness about the facts on AIDS

Successful AIDS prevention programs seek to meet real needs that are felt by the population to be served. There is a difference between the needs of the community to be served and the needs identified by health professionals. AIDS education program planners will be most effective if they understand the population as it really is.

Any program designed to reduce the risk of HIV infection must first clearly identify the target population to be served. This identification process must go beyond a simple list of risk factors. Instead, it is best when drawn from an indepth understanding of the group members for whom risk-reduction services are intended. The lessons gained from this process assist in the identification of community residents at risk of HIV infection and those in need of AIDS education services. Additionally, the lessons gained will help in the development of prevention programs that the community will find relevant, realistic and acceptable.

Just as knowledge by itself is not sufficient to produce behavior change, the mere provision of risk-reduction services does not guarantee that they will be accepted by intended groups in the community. An honest effort must be made to provide AIDS prevention services that members of the community will perceive as beneficial from their own perspective.

Methods for the Assessment of Need

Educators must carefully select their methods for needs assessment so that appropriate educational interventions may be developed. Four basic steps are involved in this process of "diagnosis":

1   Gather the data from available sources, and consolidate with new data for planning purposes. This data should include information on both the problem and the population.

2   Before planning programs, review all existing literature on the specific problems identified.

3   Survey available resources in the community to avoid overlap and to identify individuals in the community with prior experience of the problem or solutions to the problem.

4   Bring in national or state health agencies as consultants where specific data, literature, resources or experience are lacking.

The population in need of risk-reduction services is usually estimated from census data or from previous counts (e.g., the number of residents in an apartment complex). These counts must then be qualified by some exclusion criteria (i.e., ways to target which populations to include and which to exclude for service delivery). For example, some AIDS risk-reduction programs might only work with sexually active adults, or men who have sex with other men, or sex partners of intravenous drug users.

People who have participated in AIDS prevention program planning committees often complain that so much is unknown that their job is close to impossible. No matter what they do, someone or some group will be offended. This chapter will not make their job easy; however, there are a number of information-gathering techniques that can reduce some of the confusion. Sources of information that have proved useful include, but are not limited to:

▲ Population data relevant to risk factors for HIV infection

▲ Review of service utilization records

▲ Surveys of key informants (i.e., knowledgeable people in the community)

▲ Community resident surveys
  • baseline AIDS knowledge, attitude and behavior surveys
  • baseline market surveys to determine time, location
  • packaging preferences

These are further explained below.

Selected Sources of Population Data

Population data relevant to risk factors for HIV infection are available from several sources:

▲ The U.S. Bureau of Census

▲ Centers for Disease Control
  • *HIV/AIDS Surveillance Report*
  • *Morbidity and Mortality Weekly Report*
  • *Monthly Vital Statistics Report*

▲ U.S. Office of the Assistant Secretary for Health, Office of Minority Health
  • Secretary's Task Force on Black and Minority Health (eight volumes)

▲ National Center for Health Statistics
  • The National Health Interview Survey
  • Provisional Data on AIDS Knowledge, Attitudes and Beliefs

▲ National Institutes on Drug Abuse
  • National High School Drug Use Survey
  • Drug Abuse Warning Network

Census data represent the most common source. Some of the items on census surveys are relevant to AIDS education program planning. There are several advantages to the use of census data. They are considered: reliable and valid, public when in summary form, and relatively inexpensive.

Another important source of secondary data is the Centers for Disease Control. The population data and AIDS case data described in Table 1 is an example of how secondary data sources may be used to estimate need. Information in Table 1 was part of the needs assessment study utilized by the Centers for Disease Control in a plan to expand AIDS education programs into ethnic communities in the United States.

By comparing these national data with similar information at the local level, the extent of need could be estimated. At the local level, other possible sources for demographic and health-related data are: government agencies, hospitals, clinics and practitioners, school systems, police, counseling centers, business and industries, health-related voluntary agencies, planning groups and insurance companies.

Table 1

AIDS Cases in the United States by Race/Ethnicity Compared with U.S. Population

Race/Ethnicity U.S. Population	Percentage of AIDS Cases	Percentage of U.S.
White	60%	80%
Black	27%	11.5%
Hispanic	15%	6.4%
Women		
White	29%	83.5%
Black	55%	11%
Hispanic	16%	5.5%
Children		
White	23.7%	76.3%
Black	55.1%	14.6%
Hispanic	21.2%	9.1%

Based on 1980 U.S. Census figures. Items may not total to 100% due to rounding error.

A Review of Service Utilization Records

Before launching a new AIDS education program, the planning committee should take an inventory of existing agencies in the area that offer similar or related services. Such a survey will help to avoid the duplication of services and to locate **key informants** who can provide good estimates of certain community needs. For example, approximately 95% of reported AIDS cases are directly related to sexual behavior, drug use behavior and the combination of both sexual and drug use behavior. Consequently, drug treatment and prevention programs along with clinics for sexually transmitted disease and pregnancy care would have staff who could serve as key informants in plans for development of AIDS risk-reduction programs.

Surveys of Key Informants

The key informant approach involves collecting information from individuals who are considered to be experts or representatives of certain groups in the community. Key informants must be able to identify and define community needs relevant to a given topic area. An extension of this technique is to conduct focus groups of several key informants to discuss AIDS risk-reduction issues and health education needs.

Facilities and personnel currently offering a service related to risk factors for HIV infection should be identified so that an empirical study of the number of people who are being treated or served can be conducted. There are at least two approaches to determining the number of people under treatment. The most direct approach would be to survey the appropriate individuals in the target community. Physicians and counselors could be asked how may people they have served during the last 12 months who may have risk factors for HIV infection. The risk factor list would be kept short because classifying people into a few categories would be less subject to error. Additionally, gross age categories may also be used. For example, a key informant need survey may ask how many people between the ages of 10 to 17 and 18 to 64 are sexually active, use any psychoactive drugs (including alcohol and tobacco), request services for unintended pregnancies, or request services for sexually transmitted diseases (STDs).

It is important to note that key informants, even quite knowledgeable ones, often overestimate need. Consequently, estimated needs must not be treated as actual needs. They must be validated with other systematic needs assessment tools.

Community Resident Surveys

Community residents have attitudes, beliefs and behaviors that have implications for development of AIDS education programs. If the AIDS risk-reduction program is relevant to all residents, the community should ideally be surveyed systematically to obtain a representative sample of the opinions of residents.

The AIDS educator who has a community health perspective would utilize sociological and epidemiological methods that emphasize a survey approach to data collection. Survey instruments would have structured, standardized questions with pre-established categories of response. In circumstances in which "scientific rigor" is demanded, instruments are pilot tested, validated and tested for psychometric properties in advance of administration to the target population (Green, 1986).

Obtaining a truly representative sample is difficult and expensive. To avoid a clearly biased sample, the planning committee must make a careful selection of community respondents. A survey of only professionals or only low-income residents may render results useless. One approach would be to survey intact groups. Public schools and church groups are two sources of respondents that may be available to the AIDS education planning committee. Depending on the type of risk-reduction program being planned, special groups of likely service recipients could be identified. For example, AIDS education program planners would want to contact STD clinics, drug abuse treatment programs, gay and lesbian service organizations. These programs would be providing services to individuals who may be at increased risk for HIV infection (i.e., men who have sex with other men and individuals who inject drugs). Consequently, the AIDS educator could gain access to selected target populations in need of risk-reduction services.

Many AIDS education programs are designed to disseminate information to the community as a whole. Within this context, a random household survey in specific zip code areas could be used. Another approach would be a random telephone survey of selected exchanges in the target community.

Appendix A describes a needs assessment survey conducted on distinct populations in need of AIDS education. Construction of surveys requires careful planning and attention to details. It is important to keep in mind that the purpose of the survey may include, but not be limited to, a determination of:

▲ The level of AIDS knowledge

▲ Prevalence of self-reported risk behaviors for HIV infection

▲ Attitudes and beliefs that may be barriers to AIDS education efforts

▲ Acceptability of AIDS risk-reduction program components

▲ Preferences for who should deliver the AIDS education message

▲ The most convenient time and location of the AIDS education program

Summary and Conclusions

The needs assessment is the starting point for laying the groundwork for program planning and evaluation. Our determination of program effectiveness is only meaningful and useful if we have first accurately assessed needs (Green and Lewis, 1986).

Need is at best a relative concept and the definition of need depends primarily on those who undertake the identification and assessment effort. Needs are based on values, culture, past history and experiences of the individual and the community. Communities and their needs are dynamic and in a constant state of flux. The needs assessment process may occur at a single point in time to define a new program, or it may occur on an ongoing basis to reexamine priorities in light of changing needs and opportunities. Consequently, the information gathered from the needs assessment can be used to revise program goals and objectives of existing programs. The data collected in an initial needs assessment may serve as baseline measures in summative evaluation studies (Siegel, 1978; Basch, 1987). The questions in Figure 1.3 may be useful when AIDS education program planners consider conducting a needs assessment.

The end result of your needs assessment should be the determination of:

▲ Characteristics and health status of the community

▲ Characteristics of existing health care delivery systems in the community

▲ Which factors are most likely to be influenced by educational interventions

▲ Which AIDS risk-reduction services require priority

Figure 1.3

Questions to Consider when Planning An AIDS Education Needs Assessment*

1. Does it make sense to conduct a needs assessment given the amount of time and money available and the likelihood that the information obtained will be used for decision making?

2. When must the needs assessment be completed to be useful for decision making?

3. How can vested interest groups and community leaders be involved in the needs assessment?

4. Who are trusted individuals that can serve as go-betweens to reach compromise among competing factions?

5. What is the purpose and scope of the needs assessment with respect to the target population and kinds of needs to be identified?

6. Are there any existing data sources that can be used in the needs assessment?

7. Which methods will be used to collect data for the needs assessment?

8. Who will be responsible for the various tasks associated with conducting the needs assessment?

9. How will the values of the people conducting the needs assessment and the values of the target population influence the process and outcome of the effort?

10. What are the limitations of the data collected in the needs assessment?

11. How will the data obtained be integrated to rank order needs and make program planning decisions?

12. What are the ethical issues involved in conducting the needs assessment (e.g., privacy raising expectations, unanticipated adverse side effects, etc.), and how will these be dealt with?

13. How can needs assessment be planned to reflect changing needs, opportunities and constraints in the community?

* Modified from Basch, 1987

These four components provide the foundation for development of scientifically sound, ethnically acceptable and culturally sensitive AIDS risk-reduction interventions.

Bibliography

Basch, C. E. 1987. Focus group interview: An underutilized research technique for improving theory and practice in health education. *Health Education Quarterly* 14(4): 404-411.

Bausell, R. B., S. Damsrosch and P. Parks. 1986. Public perceptions regarding the AIDS epidemic: Selected results from a national poll. *AIDS Research* 2(3): 253-258.

Dever, A. 1980. *Community health analysis: A holistic approach.* Germantown, MD: Aspen Systems.

DiClemente, R. J. and C. B. Boyer. 1987. Ethnic and racial misconceptions about AIDS. *Focus: A Review of AIDS Research* 2(3): 3.

DiClemente, R., C. Boyer and E. Morales. 1988. Minorities and AIDS: Knowledge, attitudes, and misconceptions among Black and Latino adolescents. *American Journal of Public Health* 78:55-57.

Fetro, J. 1988. Evaluation of AIDS education programs. In *The AIDS challenge: Prevention education for young people,* ed. M. Quackenbush, M. Nelson and K. Clark. Santa Cruz, CA: Network Publications.

Green L. and F. Lewis. 1986. Measurement and evaluation in health education and health promotion. Palo Alto, CA: Mayfield.

Holmberg, D. 1987. Poll: 28% say keep kids at home. *Newsday* 4(33).

Posavac, E. and R. Carey. 1980. *Program evaluation: Methods and case studies.* New Jersey: Prentice-Hall.

Rossi, P. and H. Freemnan. 1985. *Evaluation: A systematic approach.* 3d ed. Beverly Hills, CA: Sage Publications.

Seltzer, R., A. Gilliam and C. Stroman. 1988. Public perceptions of AIDS in the District of Columbia: Knowledge and attitudes. Institute for Urban Affairs and Research, Howard University, Washington, DC.

Spradley, J. 1979. *The ethnographic interview.* New York: Holt, Rinehart and Winston.

Scott, G. 1987. Natural history of HIV infection in children. In *Report of the Surgeon General's Workshop on Children with HIV Infection and Their Families.* Washington, DC: Department of

Health & Human Services, No.# HRS-D-MC 87-1.

Strunin, L. and R. Hingson. 1987. Acquired immunodeficiency syndrome and adolescents' knowledge, beliefs, attitudes and behaviors. *Pediatrics* 79(5): 825-828.

Thomas, S. In press. Evaluation of community based AIDS education and risk reduction projects in the Black community. *Journal of Program Planning and Evaluation.*

Thomas, S., A. Gilliam and C. Iwrey. 1989. Knowledge about AIDS and reported risk behaviors among Black college students. *Journal of American College Health* 2(38): 61-66.

Thomas, S., A. Gilliam and C. Iwrey. 1988. Evaluation of community based AIDS education reduction programs in minority populations. National Conference on the Prevention of HIV Infection and AIDS Among Racial and Ethnic Minorities in the United States, August. Centers for Disease Control, Washington, DC.

TRESP. 1988. AIDS prevention among ethnic minorities. National Institute on Drug Abuse, National Institute of Mental Health, Contract no. 271-87-8221.

Wofsy, C. 1987. Supportive care and treatment of pediatric AIDS. In *Report of the Surgeon General's Workshop on Children with HIV Infection and Their Families.* Washington, DC: Department of Health and Human Services, No.# HRS-D-MC 87-1.

2

Using Evaluation to Develop Responsive Materials

Aisha Gilliam, EdD,
and Roberta Hollander, PhD

The purpose of this chapter is to provide health professionals who work in community AIDS prevention projects with a 6-step framework that will enable them to develop effective educational materials. This framework is designed to help assess the target population's need for educational materials, evaluate the appropriateness of existing AIDS materials, and provide a process for developing relevant materials for the target population. The chapter underscores the need to include formative evaluation techniques in the design of effective materials and programs. The case study Stopping AIDS Is My Mission (SAMM) in Appendix B further illustrates the process of the framework.

Design of Effective AIDS Education Materials

AIDS information can be presented in one or more of the following ways: lectures; films and videotapes; pamphlets, brochures, posters, flip charts and other written or printed materials; and mass media campaigns using television, radio, magazines, newsletters and other news publications. Given the broad array of educational materials, how can it be ascertained that those selected are appropriate for the target audience? Do they adequately take into account the target population's sociodemographic characteristics and the nature and extent of knowledge, attitudes, perceptions and beliefs? To what extent has the message been heard and accepted by the target audience?

Whether a message is accurate, specific and oriented appropriately toward the target group can be determined through evaluation procedures. Evaluation enables planners to decide which activities and materials work effectively and thereby lead to improved programs. Although there are many barriers to carrying out program evaluation, programs and materials that are not evaluated run a high risk of failure.

Educational materials can be assessed through formative or process evaluation, which seeks to clarify the procedures and tasks involved in development. As LeFebvre and Flora (1988) note, formative evaluation can shed light on changes in the content and delivery of programs, improve their reach and effectiveness, and thus prevent the implementation of what is likely to be an unsuccessful effort.

Although materials can also be evaluated through outcome or impact evaluation, which gives evidence of short-term and long-term effects, this chapter underscores the use of formative evaluation techniques to improve the materials development process. As indicated below, each of these types of evaluation is useful in examining AIDS educational materials.

A 6-Step Framework

In an effort to design functional, appealing AIDS materials, health professionals and community workers may find of use the following steps, which have been adapted from the World Health Organization's Series on AIDS (1989), federal materials and other sources:

1   Assess and plan around the target population's need for educational materials, and using baseline feedback from the target group, establish the goals and objectives of the program.

2   Select the appropriate AIDS education materials and channels to reach the target group.

3   As a part of concept development, conduct pretesting and revision of materials as a formative method of evaluating their relevancy and effectiveness.

4   Determine the process for production and dissemination of materials, including a method for tracking audience exposure and reaction.

5   Assess the effectiveness of the materials by studying their usage or evaluating their impact, i.e., through surveys and user logs.

6   Analyze and interpret all data collected and evaluate against initial planning and assessment for use in replanning new cycles of materials and messages.

These steps are discussed in greater detail in Figure 2.1.

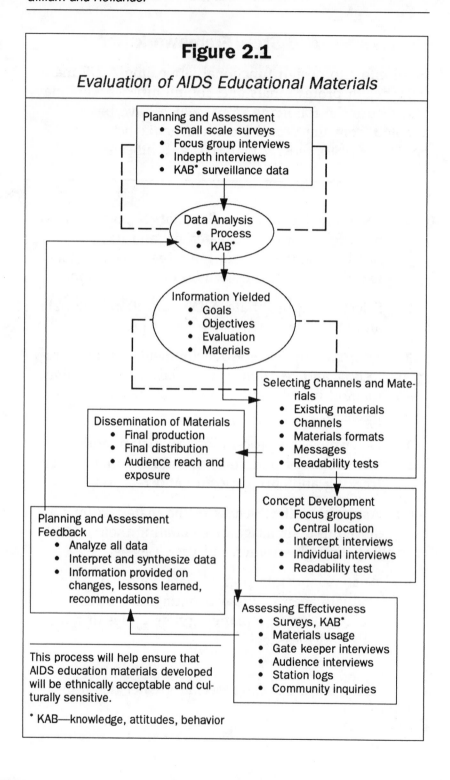

Figure 2.1

Evaluation of AIDS Educational Materials

Planning and Assessment
- Small scale surveys
- Focus group interviews
- Indepth interviews
- KAB* surveillance data

Data Analysis
- Process
- KAB*

Information Yielded
- Goals
- Objectives
- Evaluation
- Materials

Selecting Channels and Materials
- Existing materials
- Channels
- Materials formats
- Messages
- Readability tests

Dissemination of Materials
- Final production
- Final distribution
- Audience reach and exposure

Concept Development
- Focus groups
- Central location
- Intercept interviews
- Individual interviews
- Readability test

Planning and Assessment Feedback
- Analyze all data
- Interpret and synthesize data
- Information provided on changes, lessons learned, recommendations

Assessing Effectiveness
- Surveys, KAB*
- Materials usage
- Gate keeper interviews
- Audience interviews
- Station logs
- Community inquiries

This process will help ensure that AIDS education materials developed will be ethnically acceptable and culturally sensitive.

* KAB—knowledge, attitudes, behavior

Step 1: Planning and Assessment

Health communities must be premised on a clear understanding of the needs and perceptions of the target audience. Obtaining such knowledge diminishes the risk of developing irrelevant or culturally insensitive materials. An integral part of this process is to encourage ongoing feedback from the target group. This can be accomplished through interviews, focus groups and surveys or tests of level of or deficits in knowledge, as well as assessments of attitudes, perceptions and behaviors. As a result of this process, planners will be able to establish the goals and objectives of the program and select communication strategies. Specifically, small scale interviews, indepth interviews and other sources yield information about the following:

- target audience
- knowledge, attitudes and behavior (KAB)
- knowledge deficits
- goals
- objectives
- evaluation strategies
- communication strategies

Baseline data gathered at this point in the process can be compared to data from the program and at followup to determine program success (Valdiserri, 1989). In addition, this information can provide feedback for planning and strategy development in the event that changes or additions need to be made.

Step 2: Selecting AIDS Education Materials and Channels

In the second phase of material development some of the key issues to be considered are:

▲ Specification of the target group

▲ Availability and appropriateness of existing materials

▲ Appropriateness of channels for reaching the target group

▲ Materials best suited for the message, depending on whether the materials are to be used to impart factual information, increase skills or otherwise help motivate participants to reduce risks. If materials already exist which meet these needs, this is the time to evaluate and review them. This is the point at which gaps are identified.

Step 3: Concept Development

With the information gaps identified, planners can now develop the alternative concepts that are lacking in the available materials. Pretesting of materials is an integral part of this process. Pretesting prior to distribution of materials serves several purposes by helping to assess "if the materials are relevant; if they attract attention; if the message is clear and understood; if the information is retained; if the materials make the target audience feel involved in the issues; if they are acceptable in the culture; and what combinations of presenters, formats, images and text works best" (WHO, 1989:61). Pretesting can be seen as a type of formative evaluation which permits planners to assess audience reactions before producing the materials in final form. Focus group interviews, central location interviews, survey questionnaires and readability tests are all measures that can also be used in pretesting AIDS education materials. Issues to be addressed at this stage include:

▲ **Attention**—Does the message attract or hold the audience's attention?

▲ **Comprehension**—Is the message clearly understood? Are the main ideas conveyed?

▲ **Personal relevance**—Does the target audience perceive the message to be personally relevant?

▲ **Credibility**—Is the message and/or its source perceived as believable?

▲ **Acceptability**—Is there anything in the message that may be offensive or unacceptable to the target audience?

Step 4: Dissemination of Materials

Once materials have been pretested, results analyzed and materials revised as indicated, the next step in the process is to decide how and when materials should be produced, by whom and in what quantity. Finally, planners have to choose who should distribute the materials and the manner of distribution (WHO, 1989).

It is also important to prepare staff to take inquiries and arrange for an adequate supply of materials. Audience exposure and reactions are tracked to allow for changes if necessary. Questions that need to be addressed at this point include:

▲ Is the message making it through the intended channels?

▲ Is the target audience paying attention and reacting?

▲ Do the channels need to be replaced or new ones added?

▲ Are there any changes that need to be made to improve the message, materials?

Step 5: Assessing Effectiveness

The effectiveness of materials can be assessed through through evaluation of impact. This can be accomplished through studies of knowledge, attitudes and behavior (KAB) or other measurements planned in step 1 and used throughout the life of the program. Measures can be compiled through:

▲ Measures of media and materials usage

▲ Survey of media gatekeepers, members of target audience, outreach staff

▲ Review of station logs about inquiries from the community, specifically:
  • name of material
  • dates (requested, disseminated)
  • how delivered
  • number of individuals, households, agencies

Step 6: Feedback for Planning and Assessment

This sixth stage completes the process of collecting information about the audience, the message, the channels of communication and the program's intended effect, as well provides feedback for program refinement. To successfully accomplish this step, be sure to:

▲ Analyze all data collected from baseline surveys, concept testing, message testing, assessing audience reach and exposure to messages, and compiling process measures

▲ Interpret data and synthesize for replanning new cycles of messages and materials.

The 6 steps outlined above provide a framework for formative evaluation that can help identify target audiences needs and preferences, and assist in specifying goals and objectives. Furthermore, these steps represent strategies that can be utilized to test and refine materials, as well as guard against inappropriate or ineffective products. Finally, these methods serve to provide feedback for planning, implementation and process tracking. The case study, Stopping AIDS is My Mission (SAMM), provided for you in Appendix B, is an applied example of this 6-step process.

Bibliography

Amaro, H. Considerations for prevention of HIV infection among Hispanic women. *Psychology of Women Quarterly* 12:429-443.

Allensworth, D. D. and C. R. Luther. 1986. Evaluating printed materials. *Nurse Educator* 11:18-22.

Becker, M. H. and J. J. Joseph. 1988. AIDS and behavioral change to reduce risk. *American Journal of Public Health* 78(4): 394-411.

Booth, W. 1987. Another muzzle for AIDS education? *Science* 238:1036.

Braithwaite, R. L. and N. Lythcott. 1989. Community empowerment as a strategy for health promotion for Black and other minority populations. *Journal of the American Medical Association* 261(2): 282-283.

Centers for Disease Control. 1990. U.S. AIDS cases reported through December 1989. *HIV/AIDS Surveillance, Year-End Edition* (January).

Cope, N. R. and H. R. Hall. 1985. The health status of Black women in the U.S.: Implications for the health psychology and behavioral medicine. *SAGE: A Scholarly Journal on Black Women* 2(2): 20-24.

Darity, W. A., G. B. Cernda, T. T. L. Chen et al. 1989. Cancer prevention (smoking) in the Black population: A community research/intervention model. In *Minorities and Cancer*, ed. L. A. Jones. New York: Springer-Verlag.

Doak, C. G., L. G. Doak and J. H. Root. 1985. *Teaching patients with low literacy skills.* Philadelphia: J.B. Lippincott.

Flaskerud, J. H. and C. E. Rush. 1989. AIDS and traditional health beliefs and practices of Black women. *Nursing Research* 38(4): 210-215.

Freimuth, V. S. 1979. Assessing the readability of health education messages. *Public Health Reports* 94(6): 568-70.

Freudenberg, N. 1989. *Preventing AIDS: A guide to effective education for the prevention of HIV infection.* Washington, DC: American Public Health Association.

Gadsden, S. 1987. Marketing to Blacks: Toyota taps Black buying power. *Advertising Age* 58(53): S5-S6.

Green, L. W., M. W. Kreuter, S. G. Deeds and K. B. Partridge. 1980. *Health education planning: A diagnostic approach.* Palo Alto, CA: Mayfield.

Hopkins, D. R. 1987. AIDS in minority populations in the United States. *Public Health Reports* 102(6): 677-681.

Issues in world health: AIDS education—a beginning. 1989. *Population Reports* Series L, Number 8.

Kirp, D. L. 1989. Uncommon decency: Pacific Bell responds to AIFD. *Harvard Business Review* 67(3): 140-151.

LeFebvre R. C. and J. Flora. 1988. Social marketing and public health intervention. *Health Education Quarterly* 15(3): 299-315.

Leishman, K. 1987. Heterosexuals and AIDS: The second stage of the epidemic. *The Atlantic Monthly*, Feb., 39-58.

Manning, D. T. 1981. Communicating messages via print media. *Occupational Health and Safety* 5:31-34.

Marin, G. 1989. AIDS prevention among Hispanics: Needs, risk behaviors, and cultural values. *Public Health Reports* 104(5): 411-415.

Mendelsohn, H. 1975. Some reasons why information campaigns can succeed. *Public Opinion Quarterly* 37: 50-61.

National Institutes of Health. 1984. *Pretesting in health communications.* Washington, DC: Government Printing Office. NIH Publication No. 84-1493.

National Institutes of Health. 1989. *Making health communications work: A planner's guide.* Washington DC: Government Printing Office. NIH Publication No. 89-1493.

National Institutes of Health, Office of Cancer Communications, National Cancer Institute. 1989. *Making Health Communications Work: A Planners Guide* (April). Washington, DC: Government Printing Office. NIH Publication No. 89-1493.

Nitzke, S., A. Shaw, S. Pingree and S. J. Voichick. 1986. *Writing for reading: Guide for developing materials in nutrition for low literacy adults.* Madison, WI: Department of Agricultural Journalism, University of Wisconsin.

Northouse, P. G. and L. L. Northouse. 1985. Communication in health care relationships. In *Health Communication*, ed. P.G. Northouse and L. L. Northouse, 81-95. Englewood Cliffs, NJ: Prentice-Hall Inc.

Parcel, G. S., P. R. Nader and P. J. Rogers. 1980. Health locus of control and health values: Implications for school health education. *Health Values* 4(1): 32-37.

Quackenbush, Marcia, Mary Nelson and Kay Clark, eds. 1988. *The AIDS challenge: Prevention education for young people.* Santa Cruz, CA: Network Publications.

Quinn, T. C. 1989. Perspectives on the AIDS epidemic: The experience within the United States. *Bulletin of the Pan American Health Organization* 23(1-2): 9-19.

Rogers, M. E. 1983. *Diffusion of innovations.* New York: Free Press.

Rogers, M. F. and W. W. Williams. 1987. AIDS in Blacks and Hispanics: Implications for prevention. *Issues in Science and Technology* 3:89-94.

Rogers, R. W. 1984. Changing health related attitudes and behaviors, the role of preventive health psychology. In *Social perception in clinical and counseling psychology,* ed. J.H. Harvey, J. F. Maddux, R. P. McGlynn and C.D. Stoltenberg, 91-112.

Selik, R. M., K. G. Castro and D. V. M. Pappaioanou. 1988. Racial/ Ethnic differences in the risk of AIDS in the United States. *American Journal of Public Health* 78(12): 1539-1545.

Smith, A. L. 1972. Socio-historical perspectives of black oratory. In *Language, communication and rhetoric in Black America,* ed. A. L. Smith, 38-45. New York: Harper and Row.

Smith, Roger. 1988. Muhammad warns Blacks to beware "Social AIDS." *Eclipse,* Apr. 11, 6 (Black student news magazine, University of Maryland)

Thomas, S. B. (Principal Investigator) 1988. Stopping AIDS is my mission (SAMM): A community coalition model for AIDS education prevention and risk reduction in the Black community. Robert Wood Johnson Grant no. 14629.

U.S. Department of Health and Human Services. 1985. *Report of the Secretary's Task Force on Black and Minority Health: Executive Summary.* Washington, DC: Government Printing Office. No. 85-491-313/44706.

U.S. General Accounting Office: Report to the chairman, Committee on Governmental Affairs, U.S. Senate. 1988. *AIDS Education: Reading Populations at Higher Risk* (September). Washington, DC: General Accounting Office. GAO/PEMD-88-35.

U.S. Office of Disease Prevention and Health Promotion. 1984. *Aging and health promotion: Market research for public education.* Washington, DC.

Valdiserri, R. O. 1989. *Preventing AIDS: The design of effective programs.* New Brunswick, NJ: Rutgers Univ. Press.

Wallston, K. A., B. S. Wallston and B. DeVellis. 1978. Development of multidimensional health locus of control (MHLC) scales.

Health Education Monographs 6:160-170.

Williams, L. S. 1986. AIDS risk reduction: A community health intervention for minority high risk group member. *Health Education Quarterly* 13(4): 407-421.

World Health Organization AIDS Series. 1989. *Guide to planning health promotion for AIDS prevention and control* No. 5. Geneva: World Health Organization.

3

Using Focus Group Interviews to Design Materials

Joyce V. Fetro, PhD

Introduction

Focus group interviews are carefully planned interactive discussions designed to obtain perceptions about a particular topic in a permissive, non-threatening environment (Krueger, 1988). They have been used as an exploratory research technique in marketing for many years at three different points in the media production process: during concept development, during script development, and after the rough cut.

As a qualitative research technique in health education, focus groups have an unlimited potential in the development and/or revision of educational materials, the planning of new programs, the monitoring of program implementation, and the evaluation of the effectiveness of new educational materials and programs. Unlike other research techniques, focus group interviews do not attempt to quantify the characteristics of a group, but rather look at underlying attitudes and opinions of a particular group.

In materials development, they can provide indepth information about the target audiences' needs, interests, perceptions, beliefs, motivations and concerns. More importantly, they provide information about why particular groups of people think and feel the way they do. In addition, because of the group interaction process, focus group discussions with 10 individuals will generate more information, insight and ideas than 10 individual interviews.

This chapter will discuss the focus group interview as a method for designing and/or revising effective educational materials about AIDS/HIV prevention. Specifically, it will address the appropriate use of focus group interviews, the advantages and limitations of focus groups, steps for planning and conducting focus groups and procedures for analyzing and interpreting results of focus group sessions. (For additional detail about focus group interviews, see Basch, 1987; Folch-Lyon & Trost, 1981; Goodman, 1984; Higginbotham & Cox, 1979; Krueger, 1988; and Morgan, 1988.)

Appropriate Use of Focus Group Interviews

Oftentimes, educational materials are developed or revised based on assumptions and misconceptions about the needs, concerns and perceptions of particular target audiences. Focus group interviews can be a valuable tool for reducing the distance between the developers' perceptions and the target audiences' perceptions. Focus group interviews can be used during three stages of materials development.

In the **development** of new materials, after research reviews have been conducted, focus groups can provide key information about the appropriate content, language and medium necessary to reach the target audience. Initially, they can assess the level of knowledge, needs, and experience of the target audience related to HIV infection to determine the appropriate information that should be included. But they can also determine how the information should be presented. For example, focus group discussions may identify posters as a more effective way of providing information about injection drug use and HIV infection to out-of-school youth. Or they may identify underlying normative behaviors or motivations that could be addressed through the content and language in a new pamphlet about safe sex.

Existing and draft educational materials also can be evaluated using focus group interviews. In these groups, the participants are asked to share their perceptions about specific written or audiovisual materials related to HIV infection prevention.

Focus groups will provide suggestions for material revisions and future directions for development:

▲ Is the content accurate?

▲ Are the message and language still appropriate?

▲ How does the target audience receive them?

▲ Is the information conveyed effectively?

▲ If necessary, how can it be changed to make it more appropriate?

▲ If the medium uses scenarios or stories, are they realistic?

▲ Are the characters realistic?

▲ Is there a more effective way of getting the message across?

Finally, focus groups can be used to gain insights for **marketing strategies**. Where should new educational materials about HIV infection be placed so that the target audience will read them? What methods can be used to distribute these educational materials? What existing or new communication channels be used to reach the target audience?

Advantages and Limitations of Focus Groups

Before deciding to use focus groups in designing or revising educational materials, developers should be aware of their advantages and limitations (Goodman, 1984; Krueger, 1988; Morgan, 1988). These advantages and limitations should be weighed in relation to the overall purpose of the program and the available resources.

Focus group interviews offer several advantages. They place participants in a more realistic situation leading to more candid responses to questions. They are comparatively easy to conduct and relatively low in cost. They can raise unanticipated questions or issues. And they can provide results in a short amount of time.

Focus groups also have limitations compared to other techniques. Effective focus groups require trained moderators. Assembling participants is often difficult. And the moderator has less control in focus groups than in individual interviews.

Planning and Conducting Focus Group Interviews

Several steps must be completed in the planning and conducting of successful focus group interviews. They include developing the discussion guide, identifying the participants, deciding on the length and number of focus groups, selecting the location, and moderating the session. The following sections describe key elements which should be considered in each of these steps.

Developing the Discussion Guide

The first phase of the planning process involves identifying the purpose of the focus group interviews. In other words, determine who will use the information, what kind of information is needed and how the information will be used. Are the focus groups being conducted to identify the target audiences' needs for new educational materials, to obtain their perceptions and opinions about proposed content and language of the new material, or to determine different methods of reaching the target audience with information about HIV infection?

After the purposes are clarified, a discussion guide delineating broad topics to be addressed should be developed. For each topic, a series of questions should be developed and sequenced to obtain the maximum amount of information. This is not a formal questionnaire but rather a flexible guide for discussion.

Questions with yes/no answers should be avoided. Open-ended questions, such as "What do you think about...," "How do you feel about...," or "Where do you get information about..." will elicit a variety of responses and will reveal more indepth information about perceptions and feelings. Open-ended questions should be used often, particularly at the beginning of the focus group. Toward the conclusion, more closed-ended questions should be used to narrow the range of responses. Closed-ended questions include phrases like "to what extent," "how satisfied," or "how much."

Ultimately, the discussion guide will assist the moderator in making decisions about relevant/irrelevant information and in gauging time allotment during focus group sessions.

Identifying the Participants

The selection of participants is the single most important element affecting the success of focus group interviews. Four factors must be considered during the selection process.

Target Population

Participants must be representative of the target population. For example, if a pamphlet is being developed to reach Latino women of childbearing age, the composition of the focus group would be homogeneous. That is, all participants would be Latino women between the ages of 16 and 45. Since focus groups are best conducted with individuals who are similar to each other, individual sessions with Latino women should be grouped by age.

If a video is being developed to target high-risk adolescents, focus group interviews would be more heterogeneous and would include male and female adolescents from all ethnic groups. Moreover, if the video is going to be marketed to teenagers in rural, suburban and urban areas, the focus groups should have representation of teenagers living in each of those areas.

Depending on the purpose and the sensitivity of the discussion, groups may be segregated by gender, ethnicity, or any other variable that would likely to affect the honesty of the responses and the group dynamics.

Participants can be randomly selected from neighborhoods or community localities that correspond to the relevant characteristics of the target audience. Although randomization is ideal, it is more important to assure that all possible diverse opinions of subgroups are represented by the participants.

Anonymous Interaction

Participants should *not* know each other. Existing acquaintances and friendships may have pre-established leader/follower relationships that could interfere with the interactive process. In addition, individuals are more apt to share information, feelings, and personal experiences with others if they know they will not have to interact with them afterward. Participants are often recruited through listings in telephone directories. Individuals are randomly selected, called and screened to assess whether they are typical of the intended target audience. Finally, if they agree to participate, they are informed about the location and time of the session.

Setting up focus groups with students, particularly younger students who do *not* know each other, is more difficult. Students from different schools are often unable to meet at central locations in the community because of a lack of transportation. The best option is conducting student focus groups in the school setting, but selecting students from different grade levels, tracks or classes.

Number of Participants

Focus groups typically include eight to twelve individuals from the target audience. Smaller groups may not allow for sufficient interaction and will require more active participation by each individual, and thus, may exert pressure on individuals to participate. In larger groups, all participants may not have a chance to present their points of view. Less assertive individuals may sit back in agreement rather than express their perceptions and opinions. Larger groups can be more difficult to manage and keep focused on the discussion at hand.

Provide an Incentive

Participants should be offered an incentive for their attendance and input. Most often, adults are reimbursed for travel and parking expenses in addition to receiving a stipend. Many educational organizations offer free materials and books. Younger children and adolescents can also receive stipends; however, if the focus groups are conducted during the school day, monetary compensation is often replaced with refreshments.

Time Allotment

Sessions should last 1-2 hours. This amount of time is necessary for the moderator to develop a rapport with the participants and will result in more honest, candid responses. However, the session length may vary based on the participants' ages and the purpose of the discussion. For example, since children and adolescents often have shorter attention spans, focus group sessions lasting one hour will be more successful.

Initially, the number of focus groups planned depends on the complexity of the topic to be discussed, the depth of information needed to fully develop the educational material, the number of subgroups that will be targeted, and the available time, staff and funding. Most often, three or more focus groups are conducted. If the groups are homogeneous, fewer sessions are necessary. If a larger number of subgroups are being targeted, additional sessions may be required.

Overall, the number of focus groups actually conducted will depend on the quality of participants' responses and the comparability of data collected across groups. Input is usually considered adequate when additional discussions elicit no *new* information, perceptions or ideas.

In the development of some materials, multi-stage focus groups may be advantageous. For example, a series of focus groups can be conducted to explore ideas for a new educational material based on the target audience's needs and concerns. The same participants can be brought back together to elicit their perceptions about the initial draft material. The second series of focus groups can use intact groups from the first series or can mix participants across focus groups.

Selecting the Location
The location of focus group interviews can have a marked effect on participants' responses. Focus groups should be conducted in a relaxed, unstructured, permissive environment. This relaxed atmosphere will encourage more candid, impromptu responses and will result in more indepth discussions about perceptions and feelings.

Neutrality of location is important. Sessions should not be conducted within organizations or agencies that might make some participants feel uncomfortable (e.g., churches, law enforcement agencies and administration buildings).

A community meeting room that is easy to locate and accessible to all participants is preferable. If possible, comfortable chairs should be arranged around a table so that all participants can see each other. Finally, care should be taken to minimize distractions (i.e., interruptions and outside noises) that might disrupt the group process.

Moderating the Session

Before conducting focus groups, the moderator must be aware of their purpose and be well-informed about the topics to be discussed. This will ensure that discussions are relevant and moving in a direction to elicit appropriate responses to predetermined questions.

The focus group begins with a welcome to participants, an overview of the topic to be discussed, and the groundrules. The first question, "the ice breaker," is designed to allow all participants to share some information about themselves or their experiences. This question will relax participants and lead to more specific questions.

Using the discussion guide, the moderator should keep the session focused while allowing participants to respond freely and spontaneously. If new topics emerge, he/she may choose to pursue them for additional clarification and insight.

After building a rapport with more general questions, the moderator directs the discussion in an unbiased manner, encouraging participants to openly express their feelings and perceptions about the educational material. He/she must be flexible and must be able to improvise and alter the predetermined questions to ensure input from all participants. The most important factor in eliciting honest responses is the moderator's ability to listen and probe without reacting in a judgmental manner that would influence subsequent responses.

Summarizing and Interpreting Results

Although brief notes can be taken by the moderator during focus group sessions, his/her primary role is to facilitate the discussion. Since it is impossible for the moderator to accurately remember the details of the discussion for each question, most focus group interviews are recorded either by audiotape or by the written notes of an observer/assistant moderator. In either case, the presence of the tape recorder or observer should be explained before the session begins.

Focus group interviews are a qualitative research technique. Consequently, numbers and percentages are not appropriate for reporting results. Care must be taken in interpreting the results. That is, definitive statements cannot be made and conclusions cannot be generalized. Nevertheless, focus group research can provide timely information from the perspective of the potential consumer of educational materials.

After all focus groups are completed, audiotapes should be transcribed and edited to remove all irrelevant comments. The most common method used in analyzing and summarizing focus group results is content analysis. Tape transcriptions for each focus group are reviewed. For each question, significant statements are identified, cut apart, and sorted by themes. Similarities and differences in participants' responses within groups and among groups are summarized. Significant elements, trends and patterns are identified and conclusions are drawn. Direct quotations can be used to enhance understanding of the conclusions. (For more detail about content analysis, see Berelson, 1952; Borg and Gall, 1979; Holsti, 1969; and Krippendorff, 1980).

The appropriate use of focus group interviews can provide valuable information about the target audience's needs, interests, perceptions, beliefs, motivations and concerns. Additionally, utilizing focus group interviews to design materials is another tangible way that health educators can incorporate the target community into the materials development process. This can only serve to enhance the quality and effectiveness of the materials.

Bibliography

Basch, C. E. 1987. Focus group interview: An underutilized research technique for improving theory and practice in health education. *Health Education Quarterly* 14(4): 411-448.

Berelson, B. 1952. *Content analysis in communication research.* Glencoe, IL: Free Press.

Borg, W. R. and M. D. Gall. 1979. *Educational research: An introduction.* New York: Longman.

Folch-Lyon, E. and J. F. Trost. 1981. Conducting focus group sessions. *Studies in Family Planning* 12(12): 443-449.

Goodman, R. I. 1984. Focus group interviews in media product testing. *Educational Technology* 24(8): 39-44.

Higginbotham, J. B. and K. K. Cox, eds. 1979. *Focus group interviews: A reader.* Chicago, IL: American Marketing Association.

Holsti, O. R. 1969. *Content analysis for the social sciences and humanities.* Reading, MA: Addison-Wesley.

Krippendorff, K. 1980. *Content analysis: An introduction to its methodology.* Beverly Hills, CA: Sage.

Krueger, R. A., M. Fiske and P. L. Kendall. 1956. *The focused interview.* Glencoe, IL: Free Press.

Morgan, D. L. 1988. *Focus groups as qualitative research.* Beverly Hills, CA: Sage.

National Institutes of Health. 1984. *Pretesting in health communications: Methods, examples, and resources for improving health messages and materials.* Bethesda, MD: U.S. Department of Health and Human Services, Public Health Service, National Cancer Institute. NIH Publication No. 84-1493.

Patton, M. Q. 1980. *Qualitative evaluation methods.* Beverly Hills, CA: Sage.

Viladas, J. M. 1984. *The book of survey techniques.* Greenwich, CN: Havenmeyer Books.

4

Creating Culturally Sensitive Materials

Sara Olivia Garcia

Introduction

The first thing that must be said about developing effective and culturally sensitive educational materials is that one must use all the senses in the process. To hear, to see, to feel—and most important—to be able to enter into a dialogue with those you are serving so that what is created is the result of continuing flow of communication, perceptions, and information that is uncovered and discovered.

It is as if one were painting on a large blank canvas. First, the form is painted in bits of factual information from various sources which show the cultural groups represented, the languages spoken, the age range, etc.—all information that has been gathered through demographic research and community needs assessments. Then slowly the finer, more subtle tones are added, results of the focus group interviews, and other interactions, which reflect the lives and voices of the people you ultimately want to reach. The educational materials should, in the end, blend into the painting in such a way that they do not stand out as a separate entity, but are part of the whole, able to do their part, in this case, to promote the health and well-being of its reader.

Initial Preparation

Perhaps the one most important and difficult task in developing effective and culturally sensitive AIDS educational materials is the absolute necessity that health educators get their own values and judgments out of the way, while still using their professional expertise. Elementary as it may sound, the simple exercise of clarifying where one stands in terms of preferences, biases and values helps to keep from projecting these same attributes unto others. To use the analogy once more of the canvas, the paint and paintbrushes are kept clean, clear, free of murky residue.

The following questions should serve as a personal inventory to help the health educator become aware as a first step toward objectivity and developing as clear a vision as possible:

▲   What ethnic or cultural group of people do you feel an affinity for?

▲   What ethnic and cultural group or groups do you feel most discomfort around?

▲   What do you believe is the best way to teach and learn about HIV infection?

▲   What feelings rise up in you when you think about AIDS?

Knowing Your Community

The next step is a careful specification of the group to be targeted. The more precisely the target is defined, the more effective the educational materials will be.

The following questions should give you factual information on the target populations.

Demographic Information

▲ What is the ethnic background of the target population in the community?

▲ How many years have they been in the U.S.?

▲ What were the circumstances under which they came to the U.S.?

▲ What is the age and educational range of the target population?

▲ What are the languages spoken within the community?

▲ What is the level of English dominance? Other language dominance?

▲ What is the average family's educational level within the target population?

▲ How and where do most people receive messages on health education in the community?

▲ What are some of the religious institutions supported by the community?

▲ Among the churches most attended, what are some of the beliefs about health, sex, gender roles, homosexuality, and the family?

The Physical and Social Environment

▲ Where is the community in relation to other cities, towns, etc.?

▲ What is the general "tone" of the community? Is it crowded, colorful, noisy? Are there generally a lot of people in the streets?

▲ What are the characteristics of the household?

▲ Are there centers, stores or other areas where posters and other information are displayed?

▲ Is the information conveyed in graphics, color, print? (If the latter, what literacy level?)

▲ What media is most used and popular for disseminating information? (radio, cable, newspapers, *fotonovelas*, social dances, social clubs, *fiestas*, festivals—find out the times and dates of events and programs, who the audience is, and what kind of information is conveyed.)

Community Perspective

▲ How do community leaders, members, adolescents and teachers describe the community?

▲ Where are the perceived strengths of the community?

▲ What educational tools and materials have people used or are currently using?

▲ What are the recurring themes that come up in interviews, needs assessments, focus groups, etc.?

▲ Are there elderly people in the community? If so, what is their role and place?

Knowledge and Belief About AIDS

▲ Are the conceptions of AIDS as a disease clear, consistent and well developed?

▲ Do most people in the community know the origin of the AIDS virus?

▲ Are there myths that are widely accepted and believed about AIDS? What are they?

▲ In regard to AIDS, do people know:
  • modes of transmission
  • the symptoms
  • preventive measures
  • outcomes

▲ What are the feelings most expressed in regards to AIDS?

▲ Among the community people who adhere to a religion, what beliefs about AIDS are held?

Culture, Values and Beliefs

▲ What are the most common cultural values and beliefs that are apparent in talking about AIDS and sex?

▲ In talking to people, or learning about them, do you hear a willingness to change or learn? Is there a plea for help?

Using these questions and a genuine curiosity as a filter, we embarked on developing educational materials for three distinct communities: San Juan, Puerto Rico; Bridgeport, Connecticut; and Juarez, Mexico. The following is a brief chronicle of the work we did and we offer it to you with the hope that some of our insights will provide you with some tools that will enhance your work as well.

Where Is the Hope in AIDS?*

A city-block-long mural in El Paso, Texas, created by Chicano youth, depicts AIDS as a cyclone. Across the top of the painting, you can see a menacing wind approaching. There are children, young couples, a pregnant woman holding her stomach, the elderly, all represented as a community trying to escape the wind's horror. On each side of the painting is a massive figure, one man and one woman. The figures are reassuring, strong, powerful. They evoke hope.

But, where is the hope in AIDS? We believe the hope is to be found in knowledge, in what our failures have taught us, what our successes have yielded, and what our research has proven. Through the Women at High Risk for AIDS Project, EDC set out to provide educational materials to three communities where AIDS outreach workers were preparing to provide education. The project sites were San Juan, Puerto Rico; Bridgeport, Connecticut and Juarez, Mexico. The original grant had come from an outside, government agency and stated that the community workers needed training manuals. When I arrived in each community, the workers told me they didn't want manuals. So began our work together as I came to see my role as helping each project create its own tools according to its own knowledge and needs.

---

*Reprinted with permission from "Research Within Reach: Where Is the Hope in AIDS?" in *Focus on Basics* (Winter 1990), Journal of World Education, Boston, MA.

My Role

Each of the above-mentioned projects seeks to reduce the transmission of HIV infection among prostitutes, injection drug users (IDUs) and partners of IDUs. People who are used to the street culture—many of them ex-prostitutes and former drug users themselves—are trained in AIDS prevention and education and are formed into teams. Most are women, but the projects include some men. They go out into the crack houses and shooting galleries, to bars, houses of prostitution and treatment centers. They try to identify and encourage women to come to the project's center for educational workshops, support groups and counseling.

I wanted to model an empowering process with the AIDS workers that they could, in turn, use with their communities. I tried to view myself as a giver of options and a demonstration of tools, giving them some things to choose from in developing their own materials.

I brought them everything I had come across in my own work—brochures, booklets, wallet cards and posters. Even when the outreach workers evaluated these and decided they wouldn't work, the process served as a stimulus to help them think of what *would*. At times, looking at other materials gave them confidence, affirming that other communities were thinking like they were. Other times, confidence came from realizing they had ideas that would work better in their particular situations.

From there on, I acted as a facilitator who many times just reminded us of where we were and brought us back to focus. My goal was to stay *open* and enhance and develop what was already there, in each community, trying to put my own ego aside.

I saw my role, too, as helping to establish a way of talking about sexual issues. Being a Latina myself, I know that talking publicly about sex is not part of our culture. I felt justified in challenging that value because of the severity of the AIDS crisis. The task was to find a way to talk that would make it possible to be heard. My approach was to acknowledge the cultural custom in order to respect it, to apologize for what I needed to do, and to let people know the times necessitated it. Beyond that, each project used its community's own language and ways of talking in the materials they developed.

San Juan

The first site for the project is San Juan, Puerto Rico, where the language spoken is Spanish, with most people being bilingual, and where many people travel to the United States often. When I arrived in San Juan, I discovered that the staff of *Proyecto Tú, Mujer* (Project You, Woman) knew they wanted some kind of brochure or poster, some kind of informational piece that would attract people to come to the project. I discovered that they hadn't communicated about what they believed in. They hadn't really figured out their own identity or become a cohesive group yet. So it was important to first have a lot of communication, to be able to sit down and think out loud, and yet focus on the fact that something had to be produced and rather quickly.

One of the interesting things that happened was the outreach workers figuring out that they had to offer something to the women of the community. This brought on questions like, "Are we better than they are? How do we appear to them? Are we in fact inflicting our own values on them?" So it was a dialog, not just a verbal dialog but a visual one. If they had an idea for a poster or brochure, they would actually make sketches or cut something out of magazines. Looking at it they would ask, "Is that what we believe?" or "What is that image going to convey?"

I raised the question of what the staff thought women in their community needed as motivation to learn about AIDS. I had tried to model an approach to AIDS education with the outreach workers that was based on meeting people where they are and moving on from there. The workers, in turn, did the same. The staff in San Juan thought women in their community would do things for their children that they wouldn't always do for themselves. When in the end they decided on an image for their poster, they chose to include a child.

The poster, of course, was to address women, but we asked ourselves, "What will this poster say to men?" We had long discussions of whether and how to include them. A decision was finally made to include a man shooting-up in his home, where there is a woman and a child. This came about because people wanted to convey an injection drug user who has a home—a partner, a family. And then the question, "Well, should we show him shooting-up? Is that too stark?" And there were both feelings that the poster should be stark to shock a bit, but yet to soften it by having a morning scene. In San Juan, they say, *"Se va curar."* It's interesting that the word that's used for "shooting up" is *"curar,"* which means "to cure." There was a general consensus that a man goes to shoot-up in the morning, like going into the bathroom and shaving.

The poster depicts a woman who is pregnant with a small baby on the bed. The man is in the doorway, still with the apparatus on his arm and the needle in his hand. He is looking down at them, and you can see the contradiction in the harshness of the intravenous drug and the tenderness of his gaze. The caption reads, *"Un adicto puede darte muchas cosas; a ti y a tus hijos."* ("An addict can give many things to you and to your children.")

The size is small, 10" x 15", because they wanted a poster to fit in doorways and on posts. They've flooded the city with them, and the title of the project is somewhat of a password: *"Proyecto Tú, Mujer"*; it's like saying, "You, woman, this is directed at you."

Bridgeport

The goal in Bridgeport, Connecticut is essentially the same—to reduce HIV transmission among prostitutes, drug users and their partners. Once again, many of the outreach workers themselves come from these communities. The most significant difference is that Bridgeport is very multicultural. Though predominantly Hispanic— Latinos from Puerto Rico and other Spanish-speaking countries—it's also Black and Asian. Women Who Care for Women on the Street: The Bridgeport Women's Project is situated right in the area where there are many drug users. Before I arrived, the staff was in the process of thinking about the issue of testing. Although testing had not started out to be an issue for the project, they were already being called by people who wanted to find out about it, and they needed to respond.

One person from the local AIDS task force reported that there were people already coming to the public health office for the HIV antibody test. The problem was that they were not coming back for their results. The outreach workers knew immediately that it was because people were afraid.

We talked about what kinds of materials the staff needed in order to address the fear held by those who believed they might be HIV-positive. The issue of low levels of literacy came up. They immediately said, "What happens if people can't read, or they don't read well, or it's not something that's popular?" We talked about video tapes. Of course, people who are on the streets are going to find it hard to get to a VCR. Someone thought of a poster with pictures. Considering that idea helped the group realize that what they really wanted was to give people something they could hold in their hands.

The woman who was the coordinator of the outreach workers began to talk about how she imagined people felt. I interrupted her and said, "Wait a minute, Sandy. Would you tape that? What you're saying now? Would you tape what you would tell people after they took the test, the way you would say it?" And she started by saying, "Hey girl," and she kept talking.

The message is encouraging. It says, "If you go back and you're positive, then here's how you can take care of yourself." It discusses food, rest, going out for walks. It includes a Latino message which is, "You've got to listen to music, dance once in a while, eat beans and rice"—in other words, do what's yours and what makes you "you" and happy.

At the end it encourages people to come into the women's project if they want more information or just to talk. The end product, an audiotape, is available for people to take with them when they leave the testing site, in case they don't return.

Juarez

Juarez, Mexico is across the border from El Paso, Texas. The language spoken there is Spanish, although it is quite different from the Spanish in Puerto Rico. The staff of *Proyecto Compañeros* (The Partners Project) had done an initial community needs assessment before I arrived. A range of needs emerged that were not directly related to AIDS education. The strongest message the staff received was that people wanted to learn to read. As in the other communities, I arrived in Juarez with samples of various AIDS materials. In looking through the pile, the staff saw a bit of a *fotonovela* (a comic-book format popular in Latin America), and immediately said, "This is what we need here." They made a series of six *novelas,* each with a particular message, which was to become part of a literacy curriculum for the women who would come to the project.

The main character of the *fotonovela* series is Rosa, a pregnant woman whose husband, Miguel, is an injection drug user. As the series unfolds, Rosa comes to learn about AIDS from the older women in her community. Eventually she talks to Miguel and asks him to be tested. His initial response is anger and resistance. Later, thinking about his baby, he agrees to the test. Miguel goes to the health clinic accompanied by his mother and Rosa and discovers he is HIV-positive.

In order to develop the story line, the outreach workers formed a "focus group," a gathering of people whose only purpose is to hear from many people about one particular issue or project. My part in this process was to show some possibilities in the beginning and then just brainstorm with them. The process came from them; it was something just waiting to happen. The photographs were taken (right there) in Juarez, and the text was the dialect that is used there and in other border towns like Tijuana and San Diego.

My part is over and the projects continue. I see more of what happened in hindsight. The most productive moments of my work with the staff in each project were those in which my role was to ask questions and then get out of the way, believing that out of them would come the answers to what they needed the most.

I am convinced that it is the process we undertook that brought success to the messages in the poster, tapes and *fotonovelas.* The whole community can recognize that the materials come from their streets. As if by magic, it's as if the process that led to the development of the products becomes known. It's almost as if every time someone looks at the piece of work, the realization that it was created by people in their community becomes evidence of control over one's own life. This the true meaning of community empowerment.

We at EDC had initially felt that hope was to be found in knowledge that we, through our efforts with the communities, would generate. As I reflect now on these experiences, I realize that the real hope is not found in knowledge in the traditional academic sense, i.e., those of us outside a community creating knowledge from our interactions with it. Hope is to be found as the community structures its own search for knowledge, in the questions it asks, the ideas it generates and the actions it takes.

5

Developing Low-Literacy Materials

Jane H. Root, PhD

Introduction

Surely a non-reader, or even a low-literacy reader, knows about AIDS. How could anyone not know something about a topic so much addressed by all the media and so much a subject of general conversation?

But suppose you were a non-reader and had a question—how would you find the particular information you wanted to know? All those nice pamphlets and books you might encounter probably wouldn't enlighten you. You'd try to listen in on any stray information that floated by in hopes that the particular concern you had would be addressed. But if it wasn't, you'd just be out of luck. Your knowledge, at best, might be sketchy and inaccurate.

It's tough to be a non-reader. It's dangerous, too. We know that 15-20% of the general population read so poorly that they don't count on printing as a source of information. If given a pamphlet or instructions, they may fake it. Or they may forget half of what they hear, if they have no printed resource to refer to. As the information we hope to deliver to everyone is important, we must find a way to include this 15-20% of the folks most likely to be missed with our traditional materials.

This chapter will help you plan and carry out an approach that keeps this hard-to-reach audience in mind. You will learn what low-literacy readers are like; how to write for this particular group of readers; how to use pictures, drawings and other visual materials to enhance learning; and some of the alternatives to print that may be useful.

Locating the Low-Literacy Population

Educators know that there are 27-30 million adults who do not read well enough to use print as a source of useful information. These folks may be quite intelligent, may work in responsible jobs, live in your neighborhood or attend your church. They are of no particular color or age or ethnic group. You can't tell who they are by looking at them or perhaps even by listening to them. Many have devised very effective ways of hiding their disability, even from those who know them well. They are unlikely to let a health professional know that they can't read, or read so poorly that comprehension is affected.

Knowing which person is reading-disabled is a problem. There are tests that will provide a rough approximation of reading competence (e.g., the Wide Range Achievement Test (WRAT) by Jastak Associates, Inc., Wilmington, Del.), but it is difficult to first test reading when someone wants AIDS information. It is better to provide more than one way to learn what is needed. Materials that are written in more simplified ways are one approach. Audio tapes, perhaps with a written text that parallels the tape, or slides that illustrate the message, can be used. A videotaped message is possible as well. Such alternatives will be described in this chapter.

Reaching the Low-Literacy Reader

If there is a variety of appropriate and available education materials, the health provider might say something like this to a client:

"People learn in different ways and you probably know how you prefer to learn. Some folks learn best by reading, others by listening and some like to use their eyes and ears together. Here are some pamphlets and this is a tape with the same information. You may use either or both. When you have finished I want to talk with you to be sure you know what to do. You will be in charge of your own behavior but it's my job to see that you have the information you need."

When the learner is finished, you will need to ask more than, "Is there anything you didn't understand?" You will need to ask such questions such as:

▲ "For those who are sexually active, what is the best way to reduce the chances of getting AIDS?"

▲ "If you think there is a chance that you are HIV-positive, how can you find out for sure?"

▲ "How can you get AIDS?"

▲ "How old do you have to be to get AIDS?"

Conditions for Learning

Much is required in the chain of events if the communication between client and provider is to go smoothly. You will need:

• a person who wants to learn
• an information list leading to the desired behavior
• a presentation that can be fully understood by the receiver

- learner verification by a receiver—a restatement or other means to demonstrate comprehension and willingness to comply

So, let's begin at the beginning.

Locate a Person Who Wants to Learn

Health providers are so aware of the drastic consequences of AIDS that disinterest in the matter seems unthinkable. Few would disagree that AIDS information is vital, but many teens and young adults have a notion that they can beat the odds. Death has little reality when one seems far from the age where it is a common occurrence. The threat that such a calamity can happen to one so young may not be a deterrent to unsafe sexual practices or to the sharing of needles for those in the drug culture.

Personal stories from their age-mates probably carry more weight than statistics or a general statement about how AIDS is contracted. These personal stories can be simply stated on posters or in person with groups of young people who may be in the target group. TV spots may be the best way to tell your story to an audience who might then be ready for the next step. Making a TV spot is not difficult. Make an appointment with your local TV station to get their advice and see if they will record it. Most will give you the technical assistance you'll need. You may also learn of sources of spots already made which you could obtain for local use.

Many AIDS projects employ street workers in an attempt to reach drug addicts. Some, in possible defiance of the law, distribute needles in hope of cutting down on needle exchanges. This seems to be an effective way to foster dialogue and, since there is an immediate pay-off for cooperation, some behavior may be changed. Fine legal distinctions between misdemeanors and educational efforts lose their meaning in the face of the serious consequences of AIDS. Such street workers should have *simply written* hand-outs to distribute with the needles.

Consider employing those who have already contracted AIDS as ambassadors to the groups of which they may be members. These people may be the most effective channels of information to the target group. They not only convey a credible account of the possibility of HIV infection, but they have ready access to communities at risk. Such messengers also may welcome the gratification of helping others even in the face of the dire consequences that AIDS has brought to their own lives.

Create an Information List

Low-literacy readers often must struggle to learn from print. There is a limit to what they will attempt, so you need to learn that *less is more*. To get a written message into short-term memory, the reader must recognize enough of the words to transfer them into oral language. To receive the message, a complex of neural networks operates to process it. The message must then relate to the logic, language and experience of the receiver if it is to be considered for long-term memory storage. If it fails to square with what seems reasonable and possible, if it is couched in language the reader doesn't understand, or if it deals with matters clearly outside the experience of the reader, no permanent transmission will occur.

So, choose your goals carefully. They should be *behavior-oriented* and few in number—perhaps no more than three or four in a given segment of material. Let's see how this might be done on a piece of material you may be writing:

67

▲ Audience: Teenage young people.

▲ Goals:
- Say "No" to sex; that's best.
- Use a condom; that's next best.
- Don't do drugs; that's best.
- Don't exchange needles; that's next best.

Order Messages by Importance

Most pamphlets begin by explaining at some length what AIDS is. Though few teens may know the technicalities—that AIDS is a virus that attacks the auto-immune system—it would probably be hard to find a teen who doesn't know it's fatal and that it can be sexually transmitted. Since what you encounter *first* or *last* in a communication has the most chance of sticking in memory, use this important message position for something *central* to your concern.

You might want to begin with something like this: "Anyone can get AIDS! Any body fluid (blood or semen) that gets into your body from someone else's body can give you AIDS.

"Don't fool around! The safest is to say 'No' to sex. Next best is to use a condom *every* time.

"Don't do drugs! Next best is *don't* lend a needle, and *never* use someone else's needle.

"If you think you might have AIDS, get a test to see if you are HIV-positive.

"Decide to stay healthy. It's a matter of life or death!"

Use Action Verbs, Not Inferences

The previous message is pretty concise. The essentials are there and it's short. However, you are unlikely to find such materials readily available. You may have to create them yourself. Notice the verbs in that brief message: "say", "use", "lend", "get", "decide"—all *action* verbs. Just to emphasize this point, get any AIDS pamphlet you may be using, now. Scan it to see how far through the material you must read before you find the first *action* verb which refers to some behavior you want the reader to take. I have just done this with a pile of material gathered from my local AIDS Information Project. In most, the first action verb occurs about half-way through the material. In some, there is no evidence of the need for responsible action on the part of the reader at all.

If you concern yourself largely with supplying information, you are counting on the reader to draw the appropriate conclusions. This inference-making skill is often missing or poorly developed in those who do not read easily. We assume that principles should be developed first, then suitable applications can be mentioned. This is not likely to result in successful learning for people with low-literacy abilities. Any pamphlet with solid print will go unread by those who read with difficulty. Of the pamphlets I picked up, most were fourfolds on legal size paper and printed on both sides. No doubt a skillful reader will find these helpful. The audience we are seeking to reach will find them overwhelming. They will go unread.

Develop an Appealing Presentation

Much of what has just been said applies equally well here. The language must be simple. The logic must appeal to the receiver. And it must be "do-able"—it must fit within the receiver's experience.

I recently came across a three year old in a snow-filled parking lot saying softly to herself, "We don't eat yellow snow." I'm sure her mother had explained why this is so, but I heard no such justification by the three year old, although she might recall some of it if questioned closely. She just knew the rule and she was carefully honoring it. She had been convinced that the rule made sense, so she learned it and complied.

This example of "yellow snow" may suggest a way of handling the background which justifies the behaviors we recommend. We can give emphasis to the central behaviors by including them in a written message and beginning with these "rules." Then we can add substance through discussion, by an oral presentation or by videotaped messages. Getting the message through several sensory doorways clearly helps learning.

How to Write for a Low-Literacy Audience

When you have selected the three to four points you wish to make, write a message as simply as possible. Use *conversational* style. That will avoid jargon and tend to result in shorter and more vivid language. Write in *active* voice:

> **Active:** "If you don't want to get AIDS, use a condom."
>
> **Passive:** "AIDS can be prevented by the use of a condom."

> **Active:** "Pregnant women can give AIDS to their unborn babies."
>
> **Passive:** "The AIDS virus can be passed by pregnant women to their unborn babies."

> **Active:** "Drugs can mess up your brain."
>
> **Passive:** "Brain function can be harmed by the use of drugs."

Use short statements and vivid language:

Best: "Drugs are always bad news. They can mess up your brain. Don't do drugs."

Less vivid; wordy: "People who use drugs run the risk of incurring brain dysfunction. Drugs can be dangerous and their use should be avoided."

Don't be afraid to repeat a message. Find more than one way to say it. (Note the summary statements in the box at the end of this chapter, as a second way of stating what you are now reading.)

Organize your message carefully. Then guide the reader along using headers and notes in the margin, like this:

> *Remember to use a condom every time!*

or

> *Remember:*
> *use a condom*
> *every time!*

Condoms are a girl's—and a guy's—best friend. If you have sex, use a condom! Then you are less likely to get AIDS and less likely to start a pregnancy you didn't plan on. Use a condom every time. It may save your life!

Use lower case letters whenever possible. Don't use ALL CAPS for emphasis. That makes the words harder to read, for it removes the clues provided by the shape of a word—the ascending and descending letters.

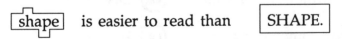 is easier to read than ┌─────────┐ SHAPE.

Key ideas can be made to stand out from the text by <u>underlining</u>, using a **bolder** type face, or by surrounding the important message with a box.

> Use a condom every time!

If there are several subjects you want to cover, or more than one audience you may want to address, consider using separate booklets rather than making a booklet bigger to cover everything. For low-literacy readers—**brief is beautiful!**

Pictures and Drawings

Now how about pictures and drawings? Pictures will aid restatement. Charts and diagrams may help if they are very simple and easily understood. However, a person with low-literacy skills doesn't learn from abstractions very well. So it is important to avoid things like a diagram of the human body, or a graph, or a table that would require a reader to find information in a box at the intersection of a horizontal row and a vertical column and then draw an inference from the information written in that box. Documents that display information in diagrams, graphs or tables are usually the least well-understood. Only competent readers can use those kinds of documents well.

Instead of such displays, you might consider using the international sign which **forbids** or indicates **OK**, like this:

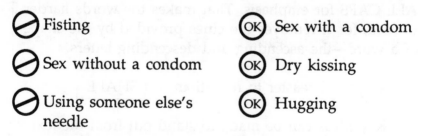

White spaces on the page, headings, and pictures with captions invite the less able reader to *try* reading;

a page full of solid print is a turn-off.

Pictures are a welcome addition. They serve to break up and humanize a text. If there is an explicit connection between a picture and the text, place the picture close to the text referring to it. If some specific part of a drawing is to be noted, call attention to it with an arrow or by putting the significant part in a different color. When appropriate, use pictures that illustrate the desired behavior.

Use high-contrast between paper and ink. Black ink on white or yellow paper has the highest contrast. Then use red, green or blue ink for adding color, variety and emphasis.

Designing Tips for Written Messages

▲ Use only 3 or 4 ideas in a section or a pamphlet.

▲ Use conversational style and active voice.

▲ Use short words and natural sentences.

▲ Use headers and margin organizers.

▲ Put important things first.

▲ Build in reviews.

▲ Use lower case letters.

▲ Leave white space on the page.

▲ Use high contrast between ink and paper.

▲ Box or underline the most important ideas.

▲ Use simple illustrations; avoid graphs or tables.

Learner Verification

You can't design *anything* that is sure to be effective without trying it out on at least a few of the people for whom it is intended. Other "experts" may add a grace note or two, but if you want the full chorus you must *find out if it works on low-literacy readers.* It's amazing how often we neglect to do this—although we'd never think of buying a car without first driving it. So, when your design is complete and includes illustrations—even if it's only produced on a copier—get at least 6 to 10 potential users to read what you have created. (Your local school system may have candidates for you in adult basic education classes, or volunteer literacy groups may be able to help.)

Design a few questions which must be answered by statements or demonstrations—not by simply "Yes" or "No"—to check on comprehension of the material which has been read. The results of a simple "pilot test" may call for a redesign. Don't let your pride-of-ownership blind you to the need for a rewrite. Health information centers are awash with pamphlets that never were subjected to this scrutiny and, as a result, many materials have been shown to be not very effective.

Before you spend a dime at the printer, also spend a few minutes "road testing" what you intend to present to the world. For some readers it may not be possible to develop written material simple enough to pass your test. You need to know if this is so, and to identify what alternative approaches it may take to inform this segment of your audience.

Alternatives Approaches

Teaching a Low-Literacy Reader with a Pamphlet

When possible, talk a poor reader through a pamphlet, pointing out the written message as you speak about it. With a felt-tipped pen, underline or circle the parts that are most significant to this particular reader. If anonymity is not a consideration, write the person's name on the front of the pamphlet. This can serve to personalize it and enhance the likelihood of a second reading and compliance.

Producing Audio Tapes

Another alternative that works well, is easily developed, and costs very little is to present the material on an audio tape. Almost everyone has access to a tape recorder. Even buying C-30 tapes at retail, you can get two or three for a dollar if you watch for sales. High-quality tapes used for music are not needed. You may be able to get a commercial recording studio to reproduce your tapes as an in-kind donation or perhaps you can get some electronics buff to show you how to reproduce tapes from one recorder to another.

You may want to talk your way through a simple pamphlet, much as you would if it was a face-to-face interaction. I would not recommend reading the material verbatim. A slight mistake here and there, a pause or even a bit of environmental noise isn't detrimental. Actually, it may well add to the natural quality of the tape. Recording two people in a dialogue or using a question and answer format may make a very effective product. Experiment a little and don't be afraid of a mistake or two.

Tapes should be no longer than six to eight minutes; shorter is better. Build in some questions for the listener as you go along. You can suggest that the tape recorder be shut off while the listener supplies the answer—either by a little personal muttering of the answer or by marking a supplied answer sheet. When the listener returns to the tape, supply the answer you expected. Build in the same kinds of reviews you would incorporate into written material.

Health-providing agencies often find that their waiting rooms are good listening stations for tape-delivered messages. A handy carrel with head phones and a receptionist who suggests their use may encourage many people to listen. If you can produce tapes in quantity, you may find their unit cost is not much greater than that of some of the pamphlets you distribute. A tape handed to a person leaving a clinic is almost guaranteed to be heard at least once. I'm not sure we could guarantee as much for our print materials. The cost of AIDS is so high, we can hardly ignore any possibility of getting the prevention message out no matter what the expense. You will sleep better at night knowing that your AIDS education menu contains something for all levels of reading competency.

Summary

We know that about one-third of the general public reads below the seventh-grade level, and that most health messages are written at a considerably higher level of difficulty. That adds a note of urgency to the task of producing AIDS information suitable for all. This chapter has tried to address that need.

Writing for an audience of low-literacy ability is not easy. It requires careful selection of only the most important information. If you remember nothing else from this chapter, remember to write in conversational style and in active voice. That should make your sentences short and make your presentation sound more natural. Build in review and *test before you print*.

Try your hand at tapes as well. They are a vastly underused media for health information. They are fun to make, and have been proven to be effective.

Until we get some better answers in the AIDS war, our best ammunition is an educational program aimed at prevention. As a front-line soldier you need a full array of equipment in your arsenal. Be sure the shelf for low-literacy people isn't empty. Resolve to stock it yourself with good material based on the suggestions in this chapter. Then, teach as though their lives depended on it. In truth, they do.

6

Adapting and Translating Materials

Ana Consuelo Matiella, MA

The purpose of this chapter is to discuss the usefulness and appropriateness of translations, the process of adapting translations and English materials, some criteria to keep in mind when adapting or developing materials, and considerations when hiring a writer to develop materials.

Are Translations Useful?

My own personal and professional bias is that translations are often ineffective short cuts to educating already underserved populations about health issues. The task of educating underserved people about AIDS is just too challenging and too delicate to rely solely on translations. Translating AIDS education materials from English to another language is simply not enough.

All of us in the field of AIDS education know that materials are most effective in reaching the target audience when they are targeted specifically to the needs, values and motivators of the target group.

Knowing this, then, why do we still do translations? I believe we do translations because: (1) we genuinely want to serve people from the diverse language groups that are represented in our communities, and (2) we don't have the funds to develop things from scratch, as it were.

Consequently, we convince ourselves that what is important is to have the information available in the target language. At least, we say, it is a step in the right direction. I would agree that at the very least, it shows a noble intent in the right direction. Unfortunately, many atrocities have been committed in the name of good intentions.

It is estimated that one in five people in the United States is functionally illiterate (Doak, 1985). As health educators, we are aware that among third-world people, the illiteracy rate is much higher. This is an important consideration when we decide to have English language health education materials translated, since translations often raise the readability level of materials.

I would like to take this opportunity to reintroduce to you a principle that many of us former and current bureaucrats are familiar with, i.e., the Peter Principle. The Peter Principle of translations states, "Educational materials that are already written at an inappropriate reading level in English will translate and rise to an equal or higher level of incompetency."

Doing and using direct translations may enable us feel better about our jobs; they may save us materials development funds; they may satisfy our funders; but unfortunately, they aren't very useful to our target populations.

When Is It Appropriate to Translate Materials?

One of the best uses for well-written translations is to provide health professionals with didactic information to use as support materials in the educational setting.

As bilingual, bicultural health professionals, we may not know the medical terminology and its explanation in the target language; we may also need help in addressing difficult questions and issues. Most of us doing bilingual, bicultural health education first learned about AIDS in English. We may know how to express ourselves effectively in the language we were educated in, but could easily be stumped in an explanation of difficult and controversial issues in the target language.

Well-translated and written didactic materials can be used by the health educator in a variety of settings. The following are some examples:

▲ They can be used as guides during individual as well as group presentations.

▲ They can be useful to health professionals, who aren't members of the target group, who have conversational competency in the target language but need help with the terminology and in delivering more indepth information and explanations.

▲ They can be useful as support materials when being interviewed on the radio or TV, since during media interviews, we seldom have the benefit of reciprocal communication and clarification.

In all of these cases, translations as support materials could help us enhance our services by providing information in a grammatically acceptable manner and helping us uphold the professional standards we strive for in any language. In the media example, they could even save us quite a bit of embarrassment.

We must acknowledge that all the services we provide are just as valuable as giving out well-written print material, that after all, print materials are support materials and that they are not meant to replace face-to-face interaction in the health education setting. But also within that context, we must question the genuine usefulness of translations as hand-out materials.

What Is the Real Issue?

Revisiting the reasons for doing translations in the first place and acknowledging our good intentions, let us now look at the issue of saving money by doing translations.

If the real reason that drives us to do translations is that we don't have the appropriate allocated funds to do the job right in the first place, then doing translations is really "settling" for less. The disenfranchised, the underserved (we know who they are) are already settling for less. Suffice it to say that we need to look closely at what we are doing as decision makers and as practitioners and question the all-too-common practice of cutting corners on the already underserved.

So if the issue is that we need to develop materials in other languages that aren't going to cost us too much money, then I propose cutting the corners someplace else.

A simply and concisely written handout with a few salient points on how to protect yourself from HIV infection is better than a three-fold, three-color pamphlet that has been inappropriately translated from a high-level English to a high-level target language. It is better to save money on paper, ink, printing, graphics, illustrations and design than to sacrifice the message by doing direct, albeit well-written translations.

What Is an Adaptation?

For the purpose of this chapter an adaptation is using material that has already been written and changing it to address the needs of the target population. There are two types of adaptations that we will briefly discuss.

One is working from a document that has already been translated from English to the target language. As we know, some translations are better than others. If you have a reasonably well translated document, (i.e., one that is at least grammatically correct and has a minimum of cultural insensitivities and biases), you can work to simplify the content and concepts and develop an acceptable educational tool.

But then you have translations from hell. These are the dissertations in disguise, the ones that find their way to your desk because they didn't work "out in the field," the ones that no one had the heart to throw away, the ones that make you regret the day you officially became linguistically competent in the target language. These are the hard ones. My advice to you is: "Avoid these."

The second type of adaptation is working from an English document, using only the content as your guide. This is the kind of adaptation you want to do. You can simplify the concepts before you start writing in the target language, thereby controlling for additional linguistic biases and assumptions.

Whether you are working with English text or an already-translated document, the first step is to analyze the material with a critical eye toward simplifying the text in the target language. Ask yourself, "Is this a book in pamphlet clothing"? Strive for no more than 250 words for a handout or simple three-fold pamphlet.

Your job and your challenge is to simplify the text and make it as concise and informational as possible.

Going now to the content information, focus on the three or four points that you consider the most important, the stuff the reader can't afford to go without. Organize this information in chunks so that the reader can easily absorb it.

Although you can run in to problems with this kind of adaptation, you can—at least from the beginning—approach the developmental process with a more sensitive and targeted effort.

After this initial analysis, you need to follow the regular materials development process and since that is what this entire book is about, some points are only briefly summarized here. I have recapped Dr. Root's developmental steps from Chapter 5. Guide yourself through the process with the following simple steps in mind:

1   Limit your objectives to 2 for each piece.

2   Use only 3 or 4 ideas in a section or a pamphlet.

3   Use conversational style and active voice.

4   Use short words and natural sentences.

5   Use headers and margin organizers.

6   Put important things first.

7   Build in reviews.

Hiring a Developmental Writer

Whether you are working with existing material in English or a translated document, one important part of this process is hiring or working with a skilled writer.

The following lists will provide you with some criteria to use when looking for a writer for your material.

Desirable Characteristics

▲ Experience and knowledge in the subject matter and in the principles of health education.

▲ Experience and skill in the target language.
  • Ask for samples of their work.
  • Check on references.

▲ Ability to write at low reading levels. This is a specialized skill. (Academically trained people often pride themselves in the manipulation of their language, yet may have problems writing simply and concisely.)

▲ Cultural identification. (Bicultural persons with specialized writing skills may have a deeper understanding and cultural sensitivity.)

Things to Clarify Before Getting Started

▲ Desired reading level and what tool or readability test will be used to assess this

▲ Specific target audience

▲ Desired style and length

▲ What the 3 or 4 major points will be

▲ How the piece will be copy edited and proofed

▲ Who will review

▲ If it will be field tested and by whom

▲ How changes will be handled

▲ Deadlines and payment

Adapted with permission from Education Programs Associates. 1989. "Translators and Translations." Campbell, CA: Education Program Associates.

This book is about the materials development process and in it you will find several discussions on the established criteria for developing effective AIDS education materials. Adaptations are not exempt from meeting this criteria.

In any educational piece, the information needs to be appropriate and relevant to the educational needs of the target population. There are no short-cuts via translations or adaptations. To strive for short-cuts is to short-change the target population.

It has been said many times that the AIDS crisis has afforded us many opportunities. One of these opportunities is the development of health education programs and materials of the highest caliber.

I encourage you to keep striving for your best in all the work you do—and don't let it stop short at translations and adaptations. As you read the rest of the book, look for the more indepth discussion of the following considerations. These are important for the development of **all** materials:

▲ Know your target group.

▲ Target as specifically as possible.

▲ Involve the target group in the design of the message and the approach.

▲ Keep readability levels low.

▲ Field test the materials before printing them.

7

Singing Your Own Song

Terry Tafoya, PhD,
and Douglas A. Wirth, BSW

Long ago, Bear invited all the other animal people to
his longhouse for Root Feast. In the old days, Indian
people of the Pacific Northwest liked to dip their food
in oil, just as you might like to put butter on your
bread or salad dressing on your salad. When the animal
people saw that there was no oil, they started to complain:

"No oil?"

"How rude!"

"Bear doesn't even know how to give a feast!"

"We should just go home!"

When Bear heard this, he laughed, being the most
spiritually powerful of the land animals. "You want
oil?" he called out, "I'll give you oil!" And he danced
out to the middle of his longhouse, singing his spirit
song, dancing to where a great fire burned, where the
salmon was roasting.

As he sang, he began to rub his great hands together over the fire. Now Bears have a lot of fat under-
neath their skin, and as he rubbed and sang, the heat of
the fire began to melt the fat, just as butter will melt
when it gets near something hot, and the fat began to
drip out in the form of oil. This was the oil that his

relatives caught in a large wooden bowl and offered to the other animal people in which to dip their food.

Now someone was watching this, and that someone was Crane. Crane envied the power and magic of Bear. The Creator had said that everyone has his or her own special song, and for many tribes part of becoming an adult is to discover your own spirit song through a vision quest, so you can become all that you can be. A song represents your potential and your behavior. The Creator said a song can be given or shared, but a song must never be stolen. Crane knew this, but he wanted the power of the Bear so badly he decided to break the law. Before the animal people left, Crane called out to them and invited them to his longhouse for a feast during the next full moon.

The people came, and it was exactly as it had been at the longhouse of Bear. There was no oil, and the people began to complain:

"No oil?"

"How rude!"

"Crane doesn't even know how to give a feast!"

"We should just go home!"

Crane laughed and he called out to the people, "You want oil? I'll give you oil!" and he danced out to the middle of his longhouse, stealing the song of Bear. He danced to where his fire was burning, and he began to rub his hands (really his feet) together as he had seen the Bear do. Now someone was watching, and that someone was the Creator. The Creator was so angry at the Crane for breaking the law, the Creator made the fire jump up, and it hit the feet of the Crane. The Crane ran away in pain and embarrassment to soak his poor, burning feet in the river, and that's where you'll still find Crane even today, still trying to cool off his burning feet.

—traditional Salish Indian legend of the Pacific Northwest

The sad reality of most exciting AIDS prevention and treatment curricula and materials is that they are designed to force everyone to sing the same song...that of a White middle-class Judeo-Christian society based on specific values and priorities. Part of the teaching of this story of Bear's Song is how the singing of a song that doesn't really belong to the singer may result in pain and damage that will last long after the last note of the song.

Beginning this chapter with a traditional Native American story is a modeling of how different societies may require alternative approaches and structuring of information than a "standard" model taught in schools of public health in dealing with sexuality and diseases like AIDS. Using existing materials and strategies without any attempt to adapt them to the targeted communities may not only be ineffective, but alienate these communities to the point that they become guarded and unwilling to accept future outreach that may be more appropriate.

In "Coyote's Eyes: Native Cognition Styles" (Tafoya, 1982), this author discusses the discipline of paradigmology. The discipline of paradigmology works from the premise that individuals and communities have vastly different interpretations of information, resulting in different ways of prioritizing what is important.

Although it may not seem evident to the mainstream culture, there are many decision-making processes that are logical and sensible.

It is a common American cultural belief and communication practice that if enough information is presented, an audience will automatically reach the same conclusion as the presenter. If the audience doesn't reach the same conclusion, the presenter will conclude the audience is resistant, stupid, crazy or hostile—or will simply provide additional information. This is analogous to turning up the oven temperature to deal with a burning cake. Increasing the intensity of individual reactions to abortion rights issues is another example of how the same "facts" lead people to different conclusions.

Indeed, just looking at the concept of priorities, one might see an AIDS prevention specialist as eagerly attempting to "convert" the public much like a neonate missionary. He/she perceives the subject of AIDS as a critical concern, especially in ethnic communities where AIDS cases continue to rise, and where, as in the case of Native Americans, sexually transmitted disease rates are considerably higher than within the general mainstream society. But the target audience may have a more critical "chain" of needs to be concerned about:

- survival/shelter
- food
- medical/dental care
- AIDS

Until the first three needs are met, there will be relatively little interest in sitting through a presentation on AIDS or reading a prevention pamphlet. This educational approach will often be perceived as boring, non-relevant, and non-respectful. This is especially true, for example, in attempting to provide services to the homeless population—a group that has been rarely addressed in AIDS concerns—and yet this audience cuts across all ethnic groups and ages.

Most AIDS educators, and educators in general, are unaware that the curriculum and materials they utilize or adapt often come with "hidden agendas" in terms of values and authority figures.

This phenomenon has also been called the hidden curriculum. The hidden curriculum is made up of the basic assumptions that lie at the foundation of the educational material or approach. Values and cultural assumptions are often rather subtle and well hidden, thus the appropriateness of the name "hidden curriculum." It is important to be aware of some of these assumptions when adapting educational materials.

Whenever you have an intercultural exchange, you will have different sets of values and assumptions operating from the different sides of the interaction. While the hidden agenda of the curriculum may indeed have some mainstream values embedded in it, the receivers of the information will also have their own perceptions that will interact. The receivers may perceive that the information was developed by an authority figure. Authority figures are almost always perceived as White male experts, so classified by their success within the White educational and socioeconomic system. This may have some obvious implications as to how effective the information will be in educating the target audience, especially if they do not recognize themselves in the authority figure's image.

Adapting and Designing AIDS Presentations

The following examples illustrate how differing values and biases can interact. All of these have implications for adapting and designing AIDS presentations and information.

Matching Appropriate Presenters and Audiences

While most AIDS education agencies (at least in terms of lip-service) recognize that it is unacceptable for the presenter to have cultural biases, the reality of dealing with ethnic communities may be that the target audience may also have some of these same biases.

In some communities, it may be judged inappropriate for a young, unmarried female to openly discuss issues of sexuality in a public forum. In other cultures, such topics as AIDS and sexuality are considered to be best talked about in gender-separated groups. While, ideally, the general American attitude would be to "convert" these "un-American" ways of acting into the ideal "egalitarian" model, the role of the AIDS prevention specialist is not to subvert generations of alternative cultural values, or to "save" only audience members who have the same values as the AIDS prevention specialist.

It is necessary for the AIDS educator to meet individuals where those individuals are, rather than where the AIDS educator would like them to be. This may require what first appear to be "non-cost-effective" approaches, such as using a team effort of "mixed" presenters, or doing the same presentation twice, once for a large female-only audience, and once for a large male-only audience, as opposed to doing one presentation for a mere handful of non-gender segregated community members.

Taking the Right Approach

A "direct" approach—"We have 50 minutes to talk about AIDS so here are the facts and statistics"—may be contraindicated with some communities. Some people of color have learning/listening styles that require an initial rapport to be established before any "facts" are discussed. To immediately begin the presentation may be analogous to a car salesperson discussing car payment options before the buyer has even been shown the car. This is one reason why stories such as "Bear and Crane" are so effective.

Storytelling

This medium provides the audience an opportunity to establish a trust relation with the presenter. In using culture-specific stories (e.g., Coyote stories for many Native American communities), audiences can be reminded of how their cultures traditionally dealt with these challenges. A point is made that this is not a "new" issue, but one that has been faced and handled successfully in the past. While AIDS itself may be thought of as a "new" disease, it is the content that is new, not the structure.

All societies historically faced concerns of sexuality, responsibilities, illness, death, abuse, etc., and have had more or less successful ways of dealing with these problems, or they would not have survived as a society. Part of the responsibility of an AIDS prevention specialist is to help empower various communities by exploring how in the past, structurally similar problems were solved.

For example, many Coyote stories of Native Americans provide an opportunity to talk about sexuality and/or abuse in a public forum. Other tribes might use Rabbit, Mink, Raven or "Culture Heroes," such as Waskijiiak, in place of Coyote—an example of how the structure can remain the same while the content changes.

Many traditional cultures place a high premium on being able to "save face," or maintain a sense of honor in public. To immediately launch into how deadly a problem AIDS can be in a specific "minority" community because of drug problems or sexually transmitted disease is to again buy into the "hidden agenda" of General America—i.e., White, middle-class society is inherently superior to "minority" communities—"You people are at even higher risk because you use drugs and have sexually transmitted diseases at a higher rate than White people." Storytelling allows topics to be brought up for discussion, but "at a distance." In other words, issues can be metaphorically addressed, because it is not an individual in the audience who is being talked about, but "Coyote," thereby avoiding defense mechanisms of denial.

Pausing for Questions

Many bilingual/bicultural communities may have significantly different presentational patterns, or respond to information in different ways. For example, there is strong empirical evidence some linguistic groups have a "pause time" that is considerably longer than that of native speakers of English. An AIDS educator who is a native speaker of English may conclude and ask, "Are there any questions?" and then pause for the standard English time of one second, which is not sufficient time to allow for some audiences to process any questions they may have. Other audiences may respond very well to modeling—an AIDS educator might conclude and say, "You know, in my experience, some audience members have some questions about..." and then list a number of actual questions that may stimulate audience members to ask the educator to give the answers. For example, the AIDS educator may mention some people want to know some very sex-specific questions that don't often get discussed—"If I come in my partner's eye, is that considered a high-risk behavior?" The very act of the AIDS prevention specialist bringing up a possibly controversial issue may provide a sense of acceptance to the audience, of subtly stating the educator is not going to be shocked by anything the audience can ask.

Choosing Appropriate Activities

"Hands-on" activities that may work very well in a

White gay setting may be inappropriate for some ethnic audiences. For example, a dildo race of putting on a condom, to see who can do it fastest, may be counter-productive for some groups such as Native Americans who do not often put a value on individualized competition, or with some Asian groups, for whom losing may indicate a loss of face. Many traditional societies which have a strong investment in "public honor" do not encourage individual members to attempt to do something in public that they have not perfected in private.

This may be very frustrating to an AIDS educator who is eager to have participants immediately begin working with condoms. It may be useful to view an activity as one that does not end upon conclusion of the presentation, but continues as the participants go home and practice with additional condoms in private. An alternative would be to use an emphasis on humor (a vital component with many traditional cultures in dealing with the learning process) to ask participants to deliberately try to use the condom incorrectly or to break it (to paradoxically discover how strong a condom is) while trying to put it on a banana, so the focus of the activity is away from trying to do an activity correctly the first time. For many people from traditional societies, competition is acceptable only within a group setting—a team competing against another team, as opposed to an individual competing against another individual.

Scheduling Presentations

In dealing with various populations, the reality is a number of presentations may have to be made. For example, it is estimated in doing outreach with the homeless, any one presentation will only reach 30% of a shelter's population. Homeless residents have different schedules. So repeat sessions must be scheduled for different times in the morning, afternoon and evening. In adapting existing materials, brochures for the homeless may be much less cost-effective than posters placed within the shelters.

Adapting and Developing AIDS Educational Materials

It is a White middle-class bias that literary materials (i.e., brochures, flyers, books, etc.) are effective outreach tools for all populations. There is a literacy problem in virtually all ethnic groups in America, compounded by concerns faced by people whose first language is not English. While culture-specific videos or *fotonovelas* may initially seem expensive as opposed to printing up a few thousand brochures, if no one responds to the brochure, it is money that has been wasted.

It is crucial to form evaluation committees that include members of impacted groups (if you're doing outreach to the homeless, you should include homeless representatives on your committee). There is also the reality that even such representatives are not perfect, and problems may arise. For example, a Native American AIDS organization published a very beautifully done poster entitled "AIDS is not a Quick Kill" illustrated with an owl, and the owl's eyes had been specially retouched to glow red. For a number of Native American groups, the owl is such a strong symbol of death it would never be publicly displayed, especially at health clinics, which were the primary intended target populations.

It is suggested that the following procedural model be utilized to insure appropriate evaluation of materials to be used in AIDS prevention:

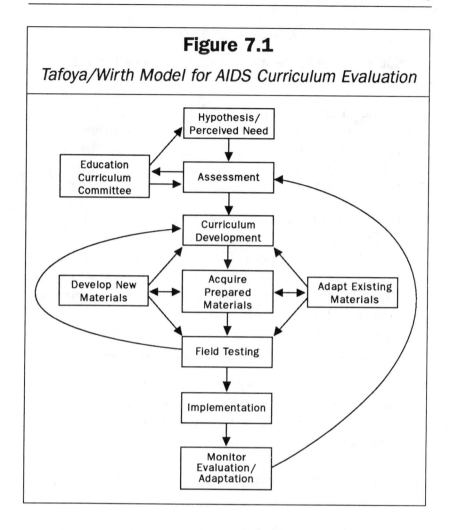

Figure 7.1

Tafoya/Wirth Model for AIDS Curriculum Evaluation

Forming an Education Curriculum Committee

In this model, it is assumed that there is an existing hypothesis or perceived need (e.g., the Indochinese refugee community is not being adequately served.) An education curriculum committee that includes members of the population being addressed should be formed.

Assessment Criteria

Assessment should be made using some of the following criteria:

▲ Is the information presented respectfully? (i.e., is there any positive aspect of the material that addresses the population, or does it deal exclusively with the dangers and problems of the community in question?)

▲ Is the information accurate? (Not just regarding AIDS—does it portray the community accurately? Are Blacks and Puerto Ricans only portrayed as drug dealers and hookers? Are Northwest coast Indians illustrated in plains Indian style headdresses? Are only historical illustrations used? For example, in doing outreach to urban Native American street youth, how realistic is it to use warriors on horses?)

▲ Does the material portray appropriate values? (e.g., Many existing AIDS curricula reflect the White middle-class bias of individualism. Curricula that stress "Do this because you can protect yourself," are much less effective in other cultures than "Do this because you can protect yourselves and your children.")

▲ Does the material/approach match the learning style of the audience? (e.g., many traditional cultures do not encourage public displays of incompetence or ignorance. It may be less effective to ask audience members to immediately demonstrate their inability to perform a task, such as putting on a condom, than it may be to model the behavior, not asking audience members to verbalize the "right" answers.)

▲ Is the material interesting? (Why bore your audience when this topic is so controversial in the first place?)

▲ Is the material at the appropriate reading level? (It is now generally known that most information on condom use provided in condom packaging is on a 12th grade reading level, or above. Should you also have available illustrations/photos that demonstrate appropriate behavior, rather than assume that a verbal/literary description is effective?)

▲ Does the presentation of the material allow for participants to ask questions or comment? (In a mixed ethnic audience, difference in pause times and assertiveness may prevent some participants from having their concerns addressed. An alternative, for example, would be the use of a talking circle—a Native American tradition in which an object such as a feather, crystal or staff is passed around in a circle, and only the person holding the object may choose to speak. This approach could radically alter the interactional style and allow every member of the group a chance to speak openly without fear of interruption or immediate criticism.

From Assessment to Field Testing

Once the education curriculum committee has been formed, the task of its members is to examine existing materials, some of which may be field tested immediately with the expectation that they are acceptable. There is certainly no need to reinvent the wheel. Other materials may require a slight or major modification to meet acceptable standards outlined in the above criteria. Still other material may be deemed totally inappropriate, and require the committee to look into the possibility of producing new material to meet the specific needs of the given population. As the model indicates, there is a continual evaluation and interaction during implementation and monitoring to permit the most effective use of resources.

It is a truism that "Good education is expensive, but bad education costs more." As was discovered in the 1970s, communities of color are not well served by taking existing curricula and darkening in the skin tones of some of the people in illustrations. A Barbie doll dyed brown is still a Barbie doll. The reality is that some of the existing AIDS curricula are simply *not* adaptable for use in all bilingual/bicultural settings. For the health of not only this generation, but generations to come, it is necessary for people to not only learn to sing their own songs, but to be permitted the opportunity to sing them.

Bibliography

Gilliland, H. and J. Reyhner. 1988. *Teaching the Native American.* Dubuque, Iowa: Kendall/Hunt Publishing Co.

Little Soldier, Dale and L. M. Forester. 1981. Applying anthropology to educational problems. *Journal of American Indian Education* 20(3): 1-6.

Scallon, R. and S. Scallon. 1983. *Narrative, literacy, and face in interethnic communication.* New Jersey: Ablex Publishing Co.

Swisher, K. and D. Deyhle. 1989. The styles of learning are different, but the teaching is just the same: Suggestions for teachers of American Indian youth. *Journal of American Indian Education—Special Issue* 1-4.

Tafoya, T. 1982. Coyote's eyes: Native cognition styles. *Journal of American Indian Education* 21(2): 21-33.

Tafoya, T. and R. Rowell. 1988. Counseling Native American gays and lesbians. In *The sourcebook on lesbian/gay health care,* ed. M. Shernoff and W. A. Scott, 63-67. Washington, DC: National Lesbian and Gay Health Foundation, Inc. (1990 edition in press)

Tafoya, Terry. 1989. Pulling coyote's tale: Native American sexuality and AIDS. In *Primary Prevention of AIDS,* ed. V. Mays. Newbury Park, CA: Sage Publications, Inc.

8

Telling A Tale

Andrea Green Rush and Dominic Cappello

Grandmother Spider
Wove the world out of herself
Silvery strands of color
Connecting all
Weaving webs of generations

Grandmother Spider, the Yuma mother and child grace the pages of *We Owe It to Ourselves and to Our Children*, a book of poetry, stories, photography and artwork. It is also a health education tool, one that uses traditional Native American storytelling and images to teach about sexually transmitted diseases (STDs). The development of *We Owe It to Ourselves and to Our Children* by the National Native American AIDS Prevention Center and Human Health Organization reflects a unique blend of health education; Native American themes, images, values, and artistic design. The book is the introductory piece to a multimedia STD and AIDS prevention package. The package consists of the *We Owe It to Ourselves and to Our Children* book and accompanying videotape and the storytelling packet.

These materials were developed to meet the need for HIV and AIDS prevention materials focusing on Native Americans and presenting information in a way that is sensitive to the values and traditions of Native American communities.

To Whom Are We Speaking?

The task of producing health education materials for Native American communities was not a simple one. The term "Native American" encompasses a diverse population that includes over 500 tribes and 200 Native villages in the United States. Native Americans live in cities, in rural communities and on reservations. Each tribe (and sometimes band within a tribe) has its own language, customs, norms, political structure, myths and legends. In urban areas there is the emergence of Pan-Indian culture, embracing people of all tribes by emphasizing the common bonds among Native Americans.

Because of this diversity it is difficult to generalize about HIV prevention education in "Indian Country." Different communities are at different points in addressing the HIV epidemic. The role of AIDS education materials in the Native American community is to open a dialogue about AIDS and to underscore that AIDS is a problem in Native communities.

We Owe It to Ourselves attempts to bridge the differences of diversity by reflecting the values and traditions that reach across tribes: the importance of the tribe, family or clan; the need for individuals to look beyond themselves to the "seven generations" to follow; the importance of survival as a people. This reflects the Native American tradition of being connected to the group, tribe or family, and it reflects the reality that STDs are not an individual problem but one of relationships and of society.

Focus group discussions have revealed that many Native Americans feel embarrassed by materials on STDs and AIDS. The issues of sex and sexuality raised by HIV infection and other STDs are considered to be very private and deeply personal in Native American communities. People do not want to be seen carrying materials with the words STDs or AIDS prominently featured. They are disinclined to pick up these materials and read them or take them home. An important part of developing the *We Owe It to Ourselves* educational materials was to make all the components of the multi-media package interesting, attractive and approachable for Native people, and to diffuse the embarrassment associated with AIDS and STDs.

Who Told the Tale

The development of *We Owe It to Ourselves* is the story of collaboration between health educators, designers, artists and storytellers. It is only through a team approach that such unique and innovative STD education materials could be developed. The initial project team consisted of Kathleen Toomey, a physician working with the Centers for Disease Control; Ron Rowell (Choctaw/Kaskaskia), director of the National Native American AIDS Prevention Center; Dominic Cappello, a health education media specialist; and Cathy Kodama, a health educator working with the University of California at Berkeley.

After conducting a national needs assessment and review of existing AIDS education materials designed for Native communities, the team concluded that there was an enormous need for all types of print and audio-visual materials. Cappello then enlisted the professional skills of designer and art director James Lambertus (Hopi), and storyteller-writer-poet-educator Terry Tafoya

105

(Taos Pueblo/Warm Springs). Key to the success of the materials is the fact that members of the targeted audience were an integral part of the team producing the materials. This underscores the most important lesson learned from the development of these materials. If a message is to be understood and accepted by a particular group of people, then they must be the ones telling the tale.

Native American health educators indicated the need for a multimedia approach that addressed a number of issues:

▲ These materials would be used in a variety of settings, from urban clinic to desert.

▲ These materials had to be uniquely Native American in design.

▲ Flexibility was vital, so that presentations could be customized to meet the needs (e.g., differing educational levels and political climates) of various tribes and groups.

Timeline for the Development Process

Over the course of 18 months, the multimedia package was developed. The following is a month-by-month timeline, outlining the developmental process:

June 1987

Kathleen Toomey, MD, meets with Dominic Cappello (designer of the video, *Sexually Transmitted Diseases: An Overview*), to inquire about the development of a video program she could use with her Native American patients. Toomey sets up a meeting with Cappello and Ron Rowell, MPH, director of the National Native American AIDS Prevention Center. A proposal is developed for production of a video program documenting the causes, symptoms, treatment and prevention of STDs (including AIDS) targeted at Native American communities.

October 1987
Secure funding for video program from Burroughs Wellcome Company. Develop and implement needs-assessment survey of 20 Native American health educators. Send out first draft of script (based on video *STDs: An Overview*) for review. Set up advisory group.

February 1988
Review needs assessment results and critique of first draft script.
Decision: In order to meet the needs of the Native American communities, all media must be distinctly Native American in graphic identity.

March 1988
Meetings with Centers for Disease Control representatives.
Decision: Video program should focus on issues related to STDs in general rather than on specific STDs and their symptoms.
Revise script (second draft). Review budget to assess possibility of developing support literature and transparencies for multi-media production. Develop video storyboard and discuss graphic imagery.
Initiate design of booklet prototype based on Native American imagery. Contract with designer James Lambertus. Content consultation with sex educator and storyteller Terry Tafoya.

April 1988
Develop first draft of education booklet (with working title *We Owe It to Ourselves and to Our Children*). Meet-

ing with Toomey, Cappello and Rowell to discuss and review first draft of booklet.

Videotape presenters and attendees at Native American Teen Conference. Note reaction of teen audience to health education videos shown. No videos feature Native Americans.

Decision: Because of teens' short attention span, video should be no longer than ten minutes. Native Americans should appear in video. Video and booklet should include imagery from at least three regions to present a Pan-Indian style rather than focus on imagery from one tribe.

Video storyboard and book prototype review by Seattle Indian Health Board and staff members. Meet with representatives from the Centers for Disease Control to present video storyboard and book prototype. Abstract describing video project selected for poster session at Fourth International AIDS Conference, Stockholm, Sweden.

May 1988

We Owe It to Ourselves and to Our Children goes into production.

July 1988

We Owe It to Ourselves and to Our Children is printed and distributed through the National Native American AIDS Prevention Center. Requests for booklets arrive weekly from both Native American and non-Native groups. Review and reassess project goals and budget.

Review the following needs identified by Native American health educators:

▲   Materials are needed that can be used with Native American health educators.

▲ Materials that can be used with overhead transparencies are as necessary as a video.

▲ Health educators need to be able to edit materials for conservative communities.

▲ Materials that educate about HIV as well as AIDS are needed in some communities.

▲ Information on caring for people with AIDS is needed in some communities.

Decision: Continue video production and begin development of storytelling packets that will include all the visuals from the video on paper (for use as handouts as well as transparencies.)

August 1988
Video storyboard and script revisions.

October 1988
25-page storytelling packet (titled *STDs: An Overview*) is developed and sent out for review.

November 1988
In response to review of packet, *STDs: An Overview*, development of an additional 25-page storytelling packet (titled *AIDS: An Overview*) begins. Review of both packets by NNAAPC training director continues. Materials used at trainings across the United States.

December 1988
Based on review by trainer and trainees, begin second draft of storytelling packets.

February 1989
Begin development of facilitator's guide for all materials (book, packets, video).

March 1989

Produce final visuals for storytelling packets and video. Produce final video script.

April 1989

Storytelling packet name changed from *Understanding AIDS* to *Understanding HIV and AIDS* to reflect greater emphasis on issues related to HIV infection.

May 1989

Select Native American video hosts/narrators. Review of materials by narrators. Tape live-action video.

June 1989

Meetings with video production technicians, computer animation specialists and art director to discuss final preparation of visuals for videotape. Produce rough cut of video (with all live-action segments and animation and visual effects). Review music (Native American flute and pipe). Review of rough cut by production team. Final production of video program.

Review of all materials by NNAAPC, members of National Education Association's Native American Caucus and San Francisco School District's media review panel. Technical assistance is provided to national distributor of entire packet, NNAAPC. Complete design of evaluation materials, forms, and mechanism for continual review and updating of materials.

How the Tale Is Told

The *We Owe It to Ourselves and to Our Children* package has three components. The first component is a book of poetry, stories and photography. Designed with flexibility in mind, it emphasizes traditional ways of speaking and can be presented orally, in the form of storytelling in a small group setting, or can simply be placed on a table or magazine rack in a clinic waiting room. Its size makes it accessible as a lap book or something to glance at while one is waiting, and its cover is inviting.

The second component is a video by the same title, narrated by two Native American health professionals. The video focuses more specifically on the prevention and treatment of STDs, HIV and AIDS. Silhouetted images are intermixed with live segments featuring Native American health educators. The eight-minute program begins with images of "Coyote," an archetypal figure, a trickster whose adventures often teach a lesson. Simple line drawings illustrate basic information. To help the health educator follow up with group discussion, the video also comes with a transcript.

The third component consists of two storytelling packets—*Understanding STDs,* and *Understanding HIV and AIDS.* Each storytelling packet includes 25 free-standing pages of all the visuals from the video, with narrative on each page. The package comes with a guide for presenters. The storytelling packets are designed to complement the video, but can also be used independently. The information in the packets can be presented orally; the images can be made into transparencies, slides for presentations, or handouts. Health educators are invited to adapt the packets to meet the needs of their audiences, to change or modify text as needed, or to rearrange the images to emphasize their particular concerns. For example, the section on condom use might not be appropriate for all audiences, and the storytelling format makes it easy for the presenter to remove the section.

We Owe It to Ourselves is effective in communicating to Native Americans because it respects and honors their sensibilities and concerns. It honors oral tradition and storytelling as important ways of communicating. It diffuses embarrassment by presenting words and images that are subtle and aesthetically pleasing. It allows the message to be presented in a way that does not affront or offend the audience.

A piece cannot communicate effectively if people do not read it and accept it, or if they feel embarrassed or offended by it. And an effective piece must come out of collaboration between people. Whether we are doctors or teachers, artists or public health workers, we are assuming the role of storyteller. And for our tale to be heard, we must engage the listener with imagination and treat our audience with the utmost respect and care.

Thanks to Ron Rowell, Doug Conway and Cathy Kodama for their assistance in the development of this chapter.

9

Producing Comic Books and Photonovels

Susan Leibtag
and Hugh Rigby

Photonovels and comic books can provide an entertaining format for learning about AIDS and other health education topics. Photographs are used to tell the story in a photonovel, and drawings are used in a comic book. Both can be very appealing to readers, particularly if they include interesting characters, an exciting plot and lively visual material.

When deciding whether comic books or photonovels might be an appropriate means of getting the message across to the intended audience, the following should be considered:

▲   Comic books and photonovels are most effective with readers who are already familiar with their formats. You could check newsstands and booksellers to see if these kinds of books are already popular with the audience.

▲   The production of comic books and photonovels requires a high level of technical expertise. It may be advisable to employ a commercial production and distribution service.

Some advantages of using comic books or photonovels for AIDS education are:

▲ Photos and drawings attract attention.

▲ Stories can hold readers' attention and be remembered.

▲ People identify with dramatic characters and will learn along with them in the story.

▲ Characters can be followed throughout a series.

▲ Real-life situations and problems, even emotional, private subjects, can be portrayed.

▲ Fantasy situations can be used for greater dramatic effect, if appropriate.

▲ Cause and effect relationships can be explained.

▲ They are popular among many age and literacy levels.

▲ A ready commercial market may exist.

▲ Corporate sponsors and advertisers are drawn to a popular medium.

The production of a photonovel or comic book is a process that involves many phases. This overview only touches upon the main principles of production. For more detailed information on the planning, production, distribution and evaluation of these materials, it is important to consult with experts in each area.

Step One: Planning

With the objectives of your project clearly defined, learn the following about your intended audience:

- levels of education/literacy, sex, age, income
- awareness of HIV infection
- main interests, questions, or preconceived ideas about AIDS
- level of visual literacy, or familiarity with understanding drawings or photographs
- familiarity with the format of comic books or photonovels
- customs and culture

Once this information is gathered, you can decide on the message to be conveyed, and on the medium (whether a photonovel or comic book). This is also the point at which to formulate a distribution and dissemination plan.

Step Two: Design

There are four basic elements of photonovels and comic books. These are **plot, dialogue, characters** and **visual content**.

Plot

The plot, or storyline, should be developed with the message woven in as a part of the story. Comics and photonovels are forms of entertainment, and are popular because the stories contain action and emotion.

In order to help the reader understand what is happening in the story, the scene changes need to be clearly marked. Present your messages as positively as possible.

Dialogue

The dialogue is the discussion between the characters of the story which takes place within the white "balloons." Dialogue consists of short sentences and vocabulary that is familiar to the reader.

Characters

The characters should be researched and developed carefully, because the personalities in your story can play critical roles in making your message understood. The audience must be able to relate to the characters in the story.

Visual Content

Attractive drawings or photographs motivate readers to pick up the photonovel or comic book in the first place. The important aspects of visual content are:

The cover. The reader sees the cover first, and then makes a quick decision whether or not to pick up the book. The cover must be interesting, and it has to compete for attention with the covers of other comic books or photonovels.

The drawings or photographs. You may want to use the type of illustrations with which the reader is already familiar. Check the popular photonovels or comic books to see what the local readers enjoy and understand. Also, be sure to pretest all visuals thoroughly.

Symbols of service delivery. These formats provide a good opportunity to tie in visuals with service delivery. You could show logos, uniforms, clinic signs, etc.

Step Three: Pretesting and Revision

Since you are trying to convey ideas and information by using pictures and words, it is important to pretest the comic book or photonovel before the final printing and make appropriate revisions to ensure that it will be effective. If possible, prepare pretest copies that look like a finished product, especially by using drawings, photographs, text and colors as they might appear in a final version. When showing the pretest you can ask:

▲   Do you like the cover?

▲ Do you like the story?

▲ Do you like the pictures?

▲ What happened in the story?

▲ Do you understand all of the words?

▲ Did you learn anything from reading this?

▲ What have you learned?

▲ Is there anything that you think is untrue?

▲ Is there anything that you find offensive?

Also, be sure that the reader can follow from frame to frame, that the action is clear and that the time sequence is clear.

Gather responses from a wide variety of individuals in the intended audience. Then you can make whatever changes are necessary to improve the book's effectiveness.

Step Four: Printing

After you have made all revisions, the comic book or photonovel will be ready for printing.

Step Five: Distribution and Dissemination

There are many different ways to distribute these types of materials. The distribution plan will depend on the audience. Photonovels and comic books can be distributed at newsstands, on public transport, in clinic waiting rooms, agency lobbies, in stores, restaurants, bars and other commercial outlets.

In some cases photonovels and comic books have been distributed to companies which have given them to employees. All available methods must be researched. Remember, it is important to plan distribution as carefully as production.

Reprinted with permission from The Johns Hopkins Center for Communication Programs. 1989. *Photonovels & Comic Books for Family Planning*. Baltimore, MD: The Johns Hopkins University, Population Communication Service.

10

Developing Relevant Materials on a Low Budget

Sala Udin

Multicultural Training Resource Center (MTRC) has been in operation as a resource center for five years. Within this time, MTRC has produced brochures, booklets, videos, manuals and posters targeting ethnic populations. We have produced materials that target African Americans and Latinos exclusively as well as multiculturally, and we have produced materials in English, Spanish, Japanese, Chinese, Korean, Cambodian, Laotian, Vietnamese and Tagalog (Filipino). We have also produced bus shelter billboards, highway billboards, bus and train cards, newspaper ads, and posters for multicultural media campaigns. *The most important lesson we have learned is that the best method of producing materials is to have the materials produced by the target community itself.*

Selecting Target Populations

Often, funding sources cannot identify the information gaps that may be targeted for certain ethnic communities. Therefore, the initial task for any material development project is to conduct a thorough survey of existing materials targeted toward a specific ethnic population to determine those information categories for which populations have been neglected, and to prioritize their information needs. Then the decision can be more intelligently made to select which specific population to target, and which particular message and issue need to be addressed for that target population.

Selecting a Format

The second kind of assessment that is required relates to the format of the material to be produced. Sometimes the format will be predetermined either by the specific requirements of the contract or by the constraints of available funds. By format we mean brochure, video, booklets, poster, etc.

Consider which traditional communication formats are popular among certain populations. For example, it is well known that in the African American community, radio, African American community newspapers, and television are popular. In the Latino tradition, *fotonovelas* are a popular format, in addition to the above. Among some Asian cultures, community news may be printed on large posters and pasted to a wall in a central area where passers-by stop to read.

An assessment needs to be made as to what kind of format is most suitable given the target population, the available funds and the contract requirements. Once the format is determined, then we can proceed to assemble the team of experts who will create the final product.

Teamwork

Teamwork is an important component and concept in the development of AIDS education materials. There are many players who must cooperate and respect each other in order for the product to have maximum quality. It is incumbent upon the agency representative responsible for developing the materials to provide clear directions regarding the specific ethnic group to be targeted, the message to be conveyed, the outcome intended, the preferred format—as well as any budget constraints—so that the expert team can go about their various tasks with the maximum amount of information.

The first few meetings to discuss the concept, the format and the approach for the product should involve several community consultants who have their fingers on the pulse of the community. By providing their perspective of the product as it relates to AIDS education and cultural appropriateness, their input can keep the entire team focused.

The sponsoring agency will also play a key role in providing the task experts with ethnic-specific background and AIDS-specific background so that the information is scientifically accurate and culturally appropriate. If the budget allows, an art director should be contracted to provide coordination and unified effort among the other team members. The art director will work closely with the graphic artist, whose task it is to develop several approaches to the design of the product. The art director and the graphic artist will then come to the agency representatives and other team members with three or four different rough approaches (mock-ups) that describe the final product to be produced.

Once the broad outline of the approach is agreed to, the graphic artist can return to the drawing board to make the rough mock-ups more specific. At this time, the writer of the copy will then know exactly how much space/time will need to be absorbed by the copy and also which direction the copy development will take. If the product will contain illustrations, the illustrator will now be able to develop a selection of illustrations that are consistent with the concept, the intended outcome and the mock-up approaches agreed upon.

Illustrators

On occasion, the product might require more than an illustrator, i.e., an artist or a cartoonist. If this is the case, then the artist/cartoonist must work closely with the scriptwriter so that the artwork or cartoon panels designed are consistent with the flow and direction of the script. Cartoon art is a specific talent at which not all artists are equally adept. Do not assume that any artist is a good cartoonist.

We discovered that the artists in the San Francisco Academy of Arts College are a talented group and a valuable resource. Both students and instructors were very cooperative in arranging for students to work on such a worthwhile project, while assuring class credit for the time and work provided. However, many of the more technical aspects of preparing artwork for professional products are still being learned by the student-artist and therefore it will be important that the student-artist be provided with expert technical direction from the art director and/or graphic artist. Students will not necessarily work for free, but will work for a reduced rate.

There are many times when we have tried to cut corners by using community artists that have not been trained in art schools or graphic artists who are self-taught. However, we have learned that this is often a mistake. There are many hidden technical skills related to graphic art that will assure the product is ready for printing without major reworking by the printer, which otherwise will increase the cost considerably. So we weren't really saving money after all; we saved it on the front end only to have to pay more on the printing end.

It is therefore important that the art director and the graphic artist have the appropriate skills and experience and can provide supervision to the illustrator and cartoonist. If the budget does not provide for an art director, an experienced graphic artist can perform the role of coordinator of all of the tasks, including preparation of the final "camera-ready" product and its delivery to the printer. It may increase the graphic artist's contract by $200 or $300, but it is well worth it.

Messenger and Message

An important component of developing AIDS education messages is consideration of the "messenger." Many professionals from diverse ethnic backgrounds believe that target populations ask themselves subconscious questions, such as: "Who is it that is giving me this message? Do I know them? Do I respect them? Do I like them? Should I receive the message they are offering?"

Therefore the agency needs to be honest and clear as to the source of the message. It is sometimes useful for the agency to show the collaborative involvement of ethnically matched consultants or other community organizations who will give the reader a sense that someone from within his or her own community or ethnic group is the messenger.

Also, the question of the "message" is important. The message could be delivered in the first person plural ("we"), or might be delivered in the second person plural ("you"). Many ethnic populations are extremely sensitive to messages delivered to them from authoritative figures on high, in second person singular or plural ("you people"). However, there is also the danger of sounding patronizing with a false first person plural ("we"), especially if the agency producing the material is not of that community or culture.

One of the most difficult problems facing AIDS/ health educators who target specific ethnic populations is their impatience with certain populations' cultural and moral standards which disallow or frown on public discussion of issues related to sex, or issues that might bring shame or embarrassment to the family, such as criminal drug use. There is also tremendous impatience with religious influence which sees the behaviors that put people at risk for AIDS as sinful.

We have learned to be respectful, humble and patient. If you cannot be direct, then it is better to let the AIDS literature be indirect, allowing the follow-up, more private discussion to be more direct. We have to meet people where they are—let them do what they are comfortable with and willing to do, and support their gradual development. More progress will be made over the course of a year than a year's worth of impatient, disrespectful interaction.

Language Translation

Many ethnic populations who speak languages other than English as their first language experience a sense of cultural domination when institutions, organizations and agencies are unwilling or reluctant to communicate to them in their indigenous language. In some cases, the ethnic populations may even be bilingual but prefer to speak or read in their own language, especially in areas as sensitive as health and sex-related matters. So it's not merely a question of whether or not people can read and write and speak English; it is a question of whether or not people would *prefer* receiving communications in the language that is culturally closest to them.

Also associated with language is the issue of vernacular. Again, it has to do with the "messenger" and the "message," and if the messenger is willing to identify and acknowledge the popular use of the language— whether English or another indigenous language—by using the most popular vernacular. This can be important, especially when attempting to communicate to young people.

Respecting Cultural Concerns

Translation represents an extremely sensitive area. In the past, translations from languages other than English have frequently been treated with second-class status. Many ethnic populations consider their language to be one of the most sacred and protected symbols and expressions of their culture. Advertising agencies and other translators who don't bother to consider some of the deeper implications of language translation often use literal translation from the English language—which when read or heard by the non-English native speaker appears to be grammatically incorrect, and culturally inconsiderate and inappropriate. Therefore, due care must be taken to assure that the broad concept is written *first* in the language in which the product will be written, rather than written first in English and translated into the second language. Then it can be translated into English for review by consultants, team members and the funding source.

Style vs. Usage

Secondly, it must be recognized that there will be wide variation of *style* and *usage*, regarding how to best structure a particular idea or concept in the non-English language. When MTRC was developing materials, we often would take a Spanish, Chinese or Korean product to one translator who would make changes which we thought were changes of structure and grammar, which turned out to be changes in style.

If the agency producing the product does not read and write in the target language, it is extremely difficult to know whether or not certain translations or usages are differences in grammar or differences in style. It is therefore important that when you take a product that is written in the indigenous language to someone to review it for translation accuracy, you request that he or she limit corrections to matters of grammar, definition and correct usage—not style. If changes in style are recommended, they should be described as such to the agency representative: "This change is a *suggested* style change and not a usage change." Obviously, changes in style can be left to the discretion of the agency representatives, whereas incorrect usage must be changed.

On some occasions, when we have taken a product to a second translator who disagrees with the usage of the first translator, we have put them in touch with each other by phone so that they can arrive at some consensus on usage. Sometimes there's a thin line between correct usage and preferred style.

Printing Special Characters

When producing materials in languages which use different characters other than the Roman alphabets used in English and Spanish (e.g., Korean, Japanese, Chinese), it is helpful to have the work printed by a printer who understands the language. Oftentimes, certain characters are omitted, or a stroke or line or dot may be added to the wrong place or on the wrong angle and can present an altogether different or even opposite meaning than what was intended. A printer might be able to catch such a mistake if the printer can read the script. This can save a great deal of time, money and embarrassment.

In 1988 MTRC produced a brochure in Chinese in which we intended to say that the reader should *not* reveal AIDS test results to his or her employer, insurance company, landlord, etc. To make "should" into "should not" requires a tiny stroke on the character. The "not" stroke was lost somewhere between the first translator, the second translator, the typesetter or the printer. The brochure was printed and 3,000 copies distributed before MTRC received feedback that we were advising people they *should* reveal their AIDS test results to their employers, etc. We had to collect all remaining brochures still in circulation, reprint and redistribute them.

Reading Level

Ethnic populations often read English or even their indigenous language at a somewhat lower level than that at which most health education literature is written. This may be due to the fact that English is their second or third language, or due to the failure of the education system. Whatever the cause, it is the responsibility of the producer of AIDS education literature to determine and meet the reading level of the target population. It is not the reader's responsibility to accommodate the producer's preferred level.

There are several methods that have been developed by reading experts to determine a person's reading level. There are also methods developed to determine the reading level of a particular piece of literature.

It has been suggested that, if feasible, producers of AIDS education materials targeting ethnic populations assess the reading level of a representative sample of the target population to determine the literacy level to be utilized in materials development.

Instructions should then be issued to writers to keep their copy within those specific literacy levels. The copy produced should also be field tested with the target population. The testing process can be time consuming, so be sure to build in enough time in the production schedule.

Ethnic Faces

If we want to communicate to the readers that we identify with them, an important and effective way might be to have the faces of the characters included in the material ethnically matched with the people with whom we are trying to communicate. However, a caution should be noted here. Frequently, there is a tendency to use the same artist to draw a number of different ethnic group faces and frequently, artists outside of a particular ethnic group are unable to capture some of the subtle nuances of facial structure. Such nuances are immediately picked up by the members of the target group who see these drawings and often feel a sense of indignation and rejection, similar to the way people feel when their language is not translated with care and seriousness. Nothing will make African Americans more angry than to see an essentially White face colored in with brown ink. Products using these methods are dooming their materials from the beginning.

Role Models

The more known about the heroes and role models important to a particular cultural group, the more accurate will be the characters used within the materials who can deliver the message on behalf of the producing agency. When Jesse Jackson, Malcolm X or Martin Luther King speak to African American people, they listen.

All ethnic groups have specific heroes or certain character types that represent important role models in their culture. It is useful to skillfully include such characters, if feasible. In cases where fictionalized characters are used, the names of the characters should be culturally appropriate. We can also use characters to include both male and female genders, and a variety of role types can be included for emphasis to make the message more effective.

Cultural Symbols

Another way of communicating identification with a particular cultural group is to know what symbols, emblems or colors may be associated with that particular ethnic group. It may be a clenched fist or a red, black and green flag for African Americans, or it may be the colors of the flag of the mother country for recently immigrated Americans. There are many symbols that can be borrowed for use in culturally relevant materials. But there is also the danger of the stereotyping pitfall. Check symbols out thoroughly by field testing them first.

Scenes

Educational materials too often ignore the "background" scenes. These reflect the buildings, the streets, the kind of commercial enterprises that are seen, the empty lots, the people hanging out on the street, the kind of clothing that is worn by the characters (major as well as ancillary characters), and gestures which are used. All of these can be used to reflect a particular cultural group (as well as a particular sub-group, class, or age group within a particular culture) in order to make the cultural match as specific as possible.

The Title

Finally comes the title. Frequently, we at MTRC wait until we have developed the concept as far as we can take it before we apply a title. Then we use the opportunity of the title to catch the attention of the casual glance. Titles should be brief, simple and catchy—and at the same time, give some indication of the cultural group that has been targeted and the content of the material. There is no systematic, scientific method we can recommend that is useful in giving a product a title. It tends to be a natural outcome of an effective process.

Choosing Cost-Effective Colors and Paper

One feature that may substantially increase the cost of printed products is the number of colors used in printing. Generally, the more colors used, the more attractive and effective the product. However, each additional color usually adds a substantial increase, because the ink must be changed on the printing press. Current technology can provide a wide assortment of color variations through a method of screening basic, primary colors so that the product appears to use several different colors, when in fact what is being used are various shades of one or two basic colors. The mixture and combination of various shades of colors to give the appearance of different color schemes is an effective and creative way to add more appeal to the product.

This was the method used to develop the color variations in the comic book *Rappin'*. *Rappin'—Teens, Sex and AIDS* (1987) is a comic book targeting youth, particularly Blacks and Latinos, to educate them about preventing pregnancy, HIV/AIDS and STDs. The illustrations and language were chosen to appeal to less literate teens, while relaying important information in an interesting and entertaining fashion. Color variations cannot completely substitute for multicolored products, but in the case of *Rappin'*, we decided to use full color only for the cover. Once people were attracted by the cover, we felt the *content* of the inside pages would keep their attention and therefore did not need the same color variation as the front cover. We have received no complaints that the comic book is less attractive or less effective by virtue of the tint that is used on the inside pages, versus full coloration.

Another cost-effective option in the case of booklets, comic books or fotonovelas is the use of a newsprint for the inside pages, instead of high gloss paper.

Review and Approval

It is usually necessary that the art director, graphic artist and the entire team come together several times with renderings, which are then reviewed by the agency, the community consultants, and perhaps focus groups, as well as representatives of the funding source, to make sure that everyone buys into the concept as well as the details, prior to final layout. This is best negotiated in the contract of all the experts up front and reiterated several times, to make sure that everyone is clear that a part of their fee requires them to attend several meetings and to make changes according to the review of the other team members and funding source.

Often, the funding source requires two or three weeks' time before approval is provided. Such approval should be requested in writing. Once the agency, the focus groups, the consultants and the funding source have made final approvals of the script, illustration, graphic art, color scheme, etc., it is useful for such agreement to be documented with the signature of the agency representative.

Frequently, ideas emerge that require the previously approved product to be changed prior to delivery to the printer. It is important that the funding source and the agency representatives clearly understand the cost implications and the scheduling modifications that are implied in such changes. If, after consideration of time and costs, the funding agency and/or the agency producing the product are willing to pay the additional cost and willing to take the additional time, then changes should be made. Otherwise, careful scrutiny of all details are important *before* final approval.

Printing

It is also vitally important that the art director and/or graphic artist be closely involved with the printer all the way through the process of printing, until delivery of the printed product. It is important that the camera-ready artwork be taken to the printer by the art director and/or graphic artist, and specific written instructions be explained to the printer regarding all technical details of color, format, etc. After the written, technical detail is provided and explained to the printer, the art director and/or graphic artist should be available for telephone or face-to-face consultation should the printer have any questions.

Finally, it is critical that the art director and/or graphic artist instruct the printer to provide an opportunity for a "blue line press check" prior to actual printing of the product. Such a press check is done by the art director and/or graphic artist, who goes to the printer to physically observe the plates, the ink, etc. and gives final approval for the product to be printed. This requirement should be spelled out in the initial contract of the art director and/or graphic artist—otherwise, they may expect to charge the agency an additional fee for such consultation and press check.

Conclusion

We have attempted to use MTRC's five years of experience to highlight some of the most important features and pitfalls of producing culturally relevant AIDS education materials on a low budget. Our emphasis has focused on the respect, celebration and utilization of the particular cultural frame of reference of a specific target population; utilization of community/student artists under the supervisions of trained technicians; and creative use of color screening, blending and the selection of paper.

11

Understanding the Production Process

Lianne B. Chong

So you need to produce a poster, brochure or flyer? Trying to produce or even print a brochure requires organization. Many of us never anticipated the amount of work, or even that the "production process" took longer than a two-week period. This brief chapter will help in organizing just that.

What is this production process? It's a phrase that describes the events and actions that transpire from just thinking about producing a brochure (the concept) to actually having it printed (solution/resolution). The following steps or considerations will be discussed in this chapter:

1   Defining the scope of work

2   Selecting a designer/copywriter/illustrator

3   Approving the budget

4   Approving the contract

5   Creating a time schedule

6   Layouts and design drafts (visual design elements)

7 Producing the mechanicals (art boards)

8 Mechanicals, or, "Are these the things I take to the printer?

9 Bluelines and color keys

10 Who has final approval over the project?

11 Printers and print bids

Defining the Scope of Work

Before you even begin to design or even think of hiring a graphic designer to help, the following questions need to answered. These questions place a parameter for the task at hand and provide a deeper understanding of the process. They also help to save time, and perhaps, money.

▲ Who is your target audience?

▲ What are the objectives? (What do you plan to accomplish?)

▲ Do you have a budget?

▲ What type of format do you have in mind? (a flyer, brochure, poster, etc.)

▲ Quantity printed?

▲ What is the deadline?

▲ Who will write the copy?

▲ Will it be produced in other languages besides English?

Once these questions are answered, you can begin to look for a designer.

Selecting a Designer

Whether you choose to design the materials "in-house" or hire a designer is a question that should have been addressed and answered prior to this stage. Budget plays an important role in whether or not you hire one. Basically, the larger the budget, the more chance of hiring a graphic designer.

However, you may ask, what does a graphic designer do that you cannot do? A designer is a professional trained to use symbols, type, pictures, photographs and the like to visually communicate information. Most have college degrees in their respective fields. Many have "hands-on experience" of the processes that may seem alien to you. They are there to aid you in producing materials. But, they come at a price. If a professional look to the brochure is desired, then by all means hire a graphic designer.

A good source that will enable you to select a designer is one who has already produced printed materials. Calling upon a fellow associate or health counselor could provide you with names and possible phone numbers of designers. If not, your next step will be to go to the yellow pages under the title heading of "graphic designers."

1   Make a list of all the designers you want to contact along with their phone numbers. Three to five names are a good start.

2   While talking to arrange an appointment with them, ask if they will reduce their rates, or have non-profit rates. Ask them for an estimate of fees and expenses, and how long it will take to produce. (This alone could eliminate seeing several designers.)

3   Plan to interview designers for approximately 45-60
     minutes. Review their portfolios. Look for sample
     art pieces: Did they solve the original objective?
     Did they show imagination in addressing the prob-
     lem? Were the pieces of the material well-organized
     and neat? Could the pieces be commercially
     reproduced?

4   Ask the designer, again, for an estimate on the
     project. Given your budget, would the designer be
     interested in the job? Has the designer had any ex-
     perience in health issues or working with non-profit
     agencies? How long will the project take? Ask any
     other questions you may have in mind. Don't be
     shy. What you may not know may take longer and
     cost you more in the long run.

5   From the interview process, begin to narrow the
     field of selection. You may want to interview them
     again. Usually, a selection is made after the first
     interview.

6   At any point in the entire process, you should be
     able to ask the designer questions regarding any
     step or process. Make it a point to ask them. Good
     communication is a must. This creates a sense of
     trust and that you and the designer are working
     together as a team. If you do not have good com-
     munication or don't trust the designer, you may
     have to select another one shortly. Or at the worst,
     working with him or her may be sheer misery.

7   If you have elected not to write your own copy,
     ask the designer to make a suggestion. You may
     want the designer to supervise the copywriter. The
     same goes for an illustrator. Why? Because it allevi-
     ates the headaches of trying to supervise people
     who are professionals in another arena. The graphic

designer works with copywriters and illustrators all the time. He/she can make suggestions, and look for those people whose style of writing and illustrating will complement the design and project. More likely, he/she will be able to coordinate the various egos involved. This will leave you to make the most important task: decision making. Overall, the process of selecting a designer should take a week.

Approving the Budget

Prior to meeting with the designer, you should have answered the question of the amount of money to be spent for the project. Have the selected designer give you an estimate for the work involved. Allow three to five working days to have this step completed.

Several items may influence the estimate:

▲   Who is writing the copy?

▲   Will the material be produced in another language? (This may require more money for typesetting.)

▲   How many colors will be used in the printing? (The more colors, the more expensive the design, production and printing will be.)

▲   The finished size of the printed piece will affect the printing cost.

▲   Are there any photographs or illustrations?

▲   Is the entire project due in less than 12 weeks? (The usual turn-around-time needed to produce a printed piece is 3 months; longer if it will be produced in other languages.) If the project is needed within, say, 5-8 weeks you may pay a premium, or a rush fee for the entire amount.

Approving the Contract

The contract is another matter that you should review closely. A contract typically is furnished along with the bid estimates from the designer. It states what the designer will be doing (scope of work), materials deadline to the designer from the client, design fee, production and print cost. It should also have terms of agreement. This should be signed by the designer and yourself as a legally binding contract. In some cases, a designer may choose to inform you of the agreement on his stationery, sent in the form of a letter.

Several items in the contract that may need clarification:

Ownership of Artwork

Most designers own the mechanicals or art boards as well as any sketches produced. Like photographers and illustrators, the graphic designer may opt to have you pay a fee and subsequent expenses to perform the work. You are paying for a usage fee. Some may have time limits on ownership, others may require you to pay additional fees for additional usage.

Revisions/Changes

Usually one to two changes in the design and typeset copy are allowed. Additional charges are subject to be billed if more revisions become necessary.

Cancellation

Many jobs, for one reason or another, never get printed.

They are "killed" during the creative or production process. If this happens, a fee, mentioned in the contract, is charged plus expenses occurred to date.

Materials Due

This indicates when materials are to be received. If you fail to give the materials to the designer by the designated date, be aware that the proposed time schedule will have to be revised.

Payment

When and how much should be worked out in advance. Standard policy for most designers is one-third up front, one-third at the completion of the art boards, and a third at the receipt of goods.

Creating a Time Schedule

Once the budget is approved by you, the designer may then submit for your approval a time sheet or a schedule of events.

To come to these dates, the designer will usually work backwards from the date desired for the finished project. A safety period, usually one to two weeks, is built into the schedule to allow for additional time that may be requested, or for some time delay in the printing/production process.

Brochures and booklets may take three to seven months to complete from initial concept to printed materials. Flyers and posters take anywhere from one to three months. Consequently, adequate time should be planned for.

Layouts and Design Drafts

Assuming that the copy has already been written and copies were sent to the designer, you should soon be looking at layouts or drafts of what the brochure will look like. During this phase of the process, all visual elements will be addressed: the size, color, type style, style of photography or illustration. The design options are presented in a comprehensive form which will represent the finished project. You should be able to distinguish the style of type and colors to be used and where the photographs and illustrations are placed.

At this point you will have to make certain decisions. You will be asked to select a design that will be produced into art boards or mechanicals for the printer. It may take anywhere from one to three revisions to get a draft of the brochure that you like. Make sure that you like it. For any reason, if you do not like it, have it changed to suit your needs. Remember, you are paying to have someone produce brochures for you. You will have to see this brochure day in and day out. And you will have to distribute and work with them for as long as you have them. As the old cliche' goes: "You get what you pay for."

Including revisions, this phase should require a maximum of two to three weeks.

Producing the Mechanicals

The design has been selected, the illustrations done; so what is left? What needs to be done next is to physically produce the artwork or mechanicals that will be used by the printer to commercially reproduce your project.

What this first entails is having the type set by a typesetter (a service in which the copy is "set" in the style, size, width and format desired). The illustrations will then be reduced or enlarged depending on the design and placed into their appropriate spaces. Everything on these mechanicals is either glued down or indicated on the boards.

You may be asked to proofread typeset copy. Approving typeset copy at this stage is much more cost- and time-efficient. Take advantage of it.

This phase takes anywhere from one to four weeks to complete.

Mechanicals, or, "Are These the Things I Take to The Printer?"

Before the mechanicals (art boards) go to the printers, both the designer and you should carefully check each one as follows:

1   Make sure all illustration/artwork/photography is properly marked.

2   Check crop marks to confirm trim size.

3   Position stats (used to indicated the cropping and size of photos and illustrations) so they are seen as they would be in the finished piece.

4   Inspect typeset copy to insure that corrections/additions have been inserted.

5   Are the type and illustrations aligned properly? Are they straight?

Bluelines and Color Keys

After the mechanicals are at the printer, bluelines (or in some cases color keys) are made as a form of a final checking system before printing takes place. Bluelines and color keys are made from negatives made of the mechanicals. These negatives are composited, then exposed to light sensitive paper or acetate overlays, in the case of color keys, to indicate the exact color matches and registration.

It is during this step that both the designer and you should carefully look over the blueline or color key to:

1   Confirm correct trim size.

2   Check the type for breaks (break-up of actual copy, i.e., dust or other material that may impair readability).

3   See if all type copy and illustrations are straight.

4   Circle all broken type, scratches or dust spots that have appeared.

5   See that the folds are in the proper places.

6   Check for correct color breaks. (Are the correct colors in their respective places? Check so that they do not get printed in other areas.)

7   Look at the positioning of the type and illustrations in case they have been reversed.

Who Has Final Approval over the Project?

You do, plain and simple. You have paid money to have a professional designer produce the job. At critical points in the process, the designer may ask for approval in various aspects of the process: selection of comprehensive design drafts, illustrations and photographs; changes and corrections made in the drafts; proofing typeset copy; final approval of the mechanicals; and approval of bluelines prior to press. Once you've given your approval to proceed, the designer is no longer responsible for any error; you have inspected the job and as the client have final say over the job. Client approval leaves you to say what is final or needs changes. If something goes unchecked or unspotted at any approval stage and you give your approval to the job, and then something goes wrong, you are at fault.

Printers and Print Bids

If you elect to supervise the print production of your project rather than have the graphic designer do so, you have some work to do before the job goes to press.

How do you look for printers? Referrals from friends or associates are important. They can recommend printers that they have used in the past, or those with whom they have good-standing relationships. If not, check the local yellow pages under the heading "printers."

Various types of printers exist: instant print shops, trade or commercial printers and specialized printers. Unless printing such items as matchbooks, boxes, computer paper or labels, business forms, tickets, yearbooks, etc., the first two printer categories are to be used.

Once you have selected a printer, visit the facilities and meet the person who will be handling your project. While visiting the print shop:

1   Confirm that the estimate is for the job you described. If at all possible, take the design/layout drafts or the actual mechanical boards to the printer to receive an accurate estimate.

2   Confirm the price and the payment schedule. Some firms require half the amount up front, with the remaining balance due on the receipt of goods.

Others are "cash on delivery" (C.O.D.). Still others may bill you on credit (net 15-30 days).

3 Confirm delivery dates.

4 Check to see if a blueline approval is all that is necessary to proceed with printing, or if a press check will be required. Press checks are done when a job in question requires exact registration and/or exact color matches are required. The press check itself requires your approval of sample printed sheets before the entire job is processed. Press checks may take the better portion of a day, depending on the project's complexity.

Selecting a Print Shop

▲ Use an **instant** print shop when:
- you have a 1-color brochure, poster or flyer (maximum size: 11" x 17"; no special folds or die cuts)
- you need a quick turn-around period (from 1-5 days)
- you need small quantities (1-3,000 copies)
- using a simple design and layout, i.e., no reverse lettering (no white letters on a black background), tints (a percentage of the color being printed—in some cases used as design elements), or bleeds (when ink "runs" off the page)

▲ Use **trade** or **commercial** print shops:
- for more than 1-color work
- if the design is more complex than just straight copy
- when you're working with unusual sizes
- if higher quality is important

Other Considerations in the Print Bid Process

▲ Paper is 25-45% of the cost of printing a typical job. Paper is sold by weight. The thicker the stock, the more expensive. Papers come in various grades:

- bond (used in inexpensive printing and photocopying)
- text or book (papers varying from 60-100 pounds), like those of stationery quality and may be coated (glossy) or uncoated
- cover (thicker than text or bond, used for covers on catalogues and booklets)
- board (a strong, stiff stock commonly used for posters)
- specialty (newsprint, carbonless, etc.)

▲ Brochures are printed on text or book stock. In some cases, bond stock is used in low-budget productions.

▲ Posters are printed on cover or board stock.

▲ The larger the quantity ordered, the lower the price per unit (i.e., 1,000 flyers may cost $75.00, or $.075 per unit, 2,000 may cost $95.00, or $.0475 per unit).

▲ The number of colors used in the project also may increase the printing budget. Black and another color is a combination commonly used. Printing it in black alone may save 25-35%.

▲ Four-color process is the most expensive. The printing cost alone makes most nonprofit budgets consider 1-2 color usage.

▲ Solid ink coverage (areas of solid colors printed on the stock) increases costs.

▲ Bleeds (when the ink runs off the page) increase costs.

▲ Is delivery included in the original cost, or will it be billed at a later date?

▲ Final size also affects prices. For unusual or larger sizes, expect to pay more for paper stock.

▲ If you have special folds, or if the job requires special cuts, these factors will also increase your print costs.

Such is the production process in an encapsulated form. It is designed to give you a brief overview and convey special considerations to various aspects of the process. This chapter is by no means designed to take the place of consulting a professional in this area.

Remember, printed material is something that you should be proud of creating. It takes time, energy and money. But more importantly, it may save someone's life.

Bibliography

Beach, M. and K. Russon. 1989. *Papers for printing: How to choose the right paper for the right price for any job.* Portland, OR: Coast to Coast Books, Inc.

Berryman, Gregg. 1979. *Notes on graphic design and visual communication.* Los Altos, CA: William Kaufman, Inc.

Craig, J. and W. Bevington. 1989. *Working with graphic designers: A handbook for editors, copywriters, art buyers, architects, promotion directors, production managers and advertising agency personnel.* New York: Watson-Guptill Publications, a division of Billboard Publications, Inc.

Dalley, T., ed. 1980. *The complete guide to illustration and design techniques and materials.* Secaucus, NJ: Chartwell Books, Inc., a division of Book Sales, Inc.

Goldsholl, M. 1987. *Inside design: A review: 40 years of work.* Tokyo: Graphic-sha Publishing Co.

Laing, J., ed. 1984. *Do it yourself graphic design.* New York: Macmillan.

Lippi, Robert. 1987. *How to buy good printing & save money: A printer's buyer's guide.* New York: Art Direction Book Company.

Minale Tattersfield & Limited Partners. 1986. *Minale Tattersfield design & graphics.* Booth-Clibborn Editions. Bethesda, MD: Direct Mail and Trade Rights, Print Bookstore.

Muller-Brockman, J. 1989. *The graphic designer and his design problem. Gestaltungsprobleme des Grafikers. Les problemes d'un graphite.* Hastings House, NY: Visual Communication Books.

Potter, N. 1969, 1980. *What is a designer: Things. places. messages.* Reading, Great Britain: Hyphen Press.

Rand, P. 1985. *A designer's art.* New Haven, CT: Yale Univ. Press.

12

Planning Outreach and Dissemination Strategies

Ruth Lopez

Congratulations! You have completed the materials development phase of your work. However, your work is far from finished. In fact, it has only just begun. Your next step is to get these materials into the community where they can help prevent the spread of AIDS.

All your hard work in developing these materials will be for naught if they languish in agency lobbies or lie around doctors' office waiting rooms. In order for your investment of time, creative energy and money to pay off, you must develop an outreach strategy that will enable you to put your AIDS education materials directly into the hands of your target population.

This chapter offers a very subjective conceptualization of how to disseminate AIDS education materials through outreach. It is by no means the only way to do an outreach campaign. It is one way based on what I have learned in three years of work with Salud Para la Gente Clinic's *Proyecto Alarma SIDA* (PAS), an HIV education and prevention program serving the rural, largely monolingual Latino community of Watsonville, California and the surrounding agricultural Pajaro Valley.

Factors that Affect
Reaching At-Risk Individuals

For AIDS prevention projects to be effective and produce lasting results, there must be a firm foundation and a solid ongoing outreach program. The following questions will help you develop an effective outreach plan:

▲ Who is the target group?

▲ Where is the best place to reach the target group?

▲ What high-risk behaviors do we want to focus on?

▲ What are the barriers to effective outreach in this community?

▲ What specific materials are going to be used?

▲ Are these materials appropriate to the target group?

▲ What are the barriers to reaching the target group?

▲ What are the community strengths that will enhance outreach?

▲ Who are the key players in the community? Who can help?

▲ How can the use of the media be maximized?

▲ What are all the possible strategies that can be used?

▲ What are the main strategies of the outreach plan?

In planning your AIDS prevention outreach program, it is important to keep in mind that community acceptance of any such a program takes time. No matter how important the education issue is, an outreach program is essentially an imposition on the target community. This is the case whether the program is administered by a governmental agency or a community-based organization.

The reality is that you are attempting to impose your agenda on people who have not asked for your intrusion into their lives.

In doing AIDS prevention work, you are asking people to examine and change their most private, possibly even secret, behaviors. This will bring to the surface emotionally charged and in many cases guilt-ridden issues. This atmosphere makes clear thinking and good judgment difficult. Therefore it is imperative that people hear your messages on many different levels and in several different settings.

For these reasons great patience and some sagacity is required to make any outreach program a success.

Essential Ingredients
for Successful Outreach

In order for any outreach project to be successful, the following elements are vital:
- community involvement and support
- reciprocal learning opportunities
- respect for tradition and values
- adaptability

Community Involvement and Support

Without the support of the mothers, lovers, sisters, brothers, fathers, spouses and friends of those community members engaging in high-risk behavior, little can be accomplished. This being the case, you must access the informal family, neighborhood and peer networks that serve to disseminate new information in every community. Potential peer educators can only be identified and recruited in an atmosphere of acceptance and support for the project.

Learning from Each Other

Doing "outreach" needs to be approached as a reciprocal learning process and needs to be presented to the community as such. As educators we need to maintain a "we can learn from each other" attitude. Without this type of attitude, outreach efforts quickly become static and ineffective.

No matter how carefully you have researched your community or how many focus groups you have conducted, you may still find that you have made some mistakes. Correcting your course of action in outreach program planning is vital to your success. A change in course is easier when you are open to learning from your community from the onset of the program.

As a case in point, when we first started PAS, we attempted to hold public forums on AIDS in migrant labor camps. These forums were not well received. Upon the advice of one of our peer educators, we halted this outreach strategy and instead tried a more personal approach by conducting informal discussions on a room to room basis. This strategy proved a much more effective means of educating this target population group.

Humility in this respect went a long way. We were willing to learn from our community and willing to change our course when we realized we were on the wrong track.

Respect for Tradition and Values

Effective outreach can only be accomplished in an atmosphere of respect for the ideas, values and traditions of the community you are attempting to reach. Your project will be negatively impacted if you offend community members by outright rejection of their ideas, values and traditions, even if you perceive them as old-fashioned or even harmful.

For example, among the Mexican immigrant population, it is not uncommon to find individuals (usually women) who give injections of antibiotics or vitamins for a small fee. They use syringes and medications purchased in Mexico. Rather than condemning this practice, we have worked to educate both the women giving the injections and the community at large concerning the need for proper needle hygiene in these situations.

This ongoing strategy is producing behavior change among the women engaged in this cottage industry. If, on the other hand, we had chosen to challenge this ingrained cultural practice, we would have run the risk of alienating these women and isolating ourselves from the community.

Adaptability

The community of Watsonville is located just a few miles from the epicenter of the devastating October 17, 1989, Loma Prieta Earthquake. In response to this tragic event, we developed an outreach strategy for HIV/AIDS prevention during the post-quake recovery period.

Community Health Outreach Workers (CHOWs) helped local residents with immediate needs (i.e., food, shelter, and clothing); and only then, after these needs were met, did they attempt to disseminate prevention messages. In this way, the CHOWs were able to maintain contact with all our target population groups throughout this chaotic and extremely difficult period.

Outreach Strategies

You have probably heard the old saying, "You can lead a horse to water but you can't make him drink." However, you may not have heard the smart *vaquero's* (Mexican cowboy) reply, *"Dale sal!"* (give him salt).

This Mexican proverb illustrates the process of effective HIV disease prevention projects. We must lead our communities to the fountain of information and skills they need to avoid HIV infection. Then we must take the process one step further and provide the salt that will make them thirsty enough to partake of the fountain of information available. The "salt" that we have used successfully at PAS is provided for you below in the form of tried and true outreach strategies.

Street Outreach

One nonthreatening way to begin your outreach is by postering the neighborhood or community you have targeted.

Outreach teams of at least two people should poster. As they do this non-threatening work, they should be alert for any interest from residents. Give posters and AIDS education materials to anyone who seems receptive. Answer any question, but do not push yourself on anyone. Take this time to establish rapport with those who do approach you.

As you become part of the community or neighborhood landscape, you will gradually be integrated into the community. Life has taught many of us a "we/they" attitude and the disenfranchised—such as injection drug users (IDUs), ethnic groups and gay men—may seem to have a stronger sense of it. We must acknowledge that is an attitude of self-protection and be sensitive to it.

This gradual approach requires patience and is a great amount of work, but can produce good results. As you become a part of the community and gain credibility, you can develop higher-profile, more direct and personal strategies such as CHOW-initiated one-on-one educational encounters and the recruitment of peer educators. This in turn can evolve into such activities as individual and informal small group sessions in which the norms and values that sanction unsafe sex and drug-using behaviors can be examined. Only then can you begin to solicit personal commitments from target group members to adopt risk-reducing behaviors.

CHOWs

Community Health Outreach Workers (CHOWs) are a key element of any effective AIDS education and prevention program. They are the people that take your message to the streets and make it real to your target population groups and the communities they live in. Here at PAS, our CHOWs actively seek out at-risk individuals and groups and provide them with HIV prevention information and materials such as bleach and condoms. They also return to the same locations on a regular basis to follow up with the at-risk people and key opinion leaders they have encountered. In this way they are able, over time, to build rapport with enough people from within our target population groups to effect behavior change.

It is very important that CHOWs be chosen, whenever possible, from the target group or groups you are attempting to reach. For example, the majority of our AIDS prevention work is with mono-lingual Spanish-

speaking agricultural workers. Therefore, we have recruited CHOWs whose first language is Spanish, who
have experience in agricultural work and who have
lived for some time in this area.

People chosen directly from your target population
will often know instinctively how to overcome barriers
to change in their community. They will also find it
much easier to approach at-risk individuals and initiate
one-on-one and small group education sessions than an
outsider. CHOWs chosen from your target population
group will also help create an atmosphere of change
and community acceptance—vital to a successful AIDS
prevention program.

In training CHOWs it is important to keep in mind
that most people teach as they are taught. Be sure to
treat CHOW trainees with respect and build on their
experience. Use clear and simple language. Make it
clear to CHOW trainees that you do not have all the
answers and that you welcome questions, constructive
criticism, and personal initiative. This type of training
will provide CHOWs with a good basis for taking your
message to the community. (For additional information
on CHOWs programs, see Appendix C.)

Community Leaders

In order to bridge the gap between mere material dissemination and actual risk reduction, you must identify
who the community leaders are. These are the people
who are respected and listened to. This group may or
may not include:
- folk healers, *curanderos, sobadores*
- neighborhood leaders
- information leaders
- public health officials
- elected officials

- physicians, nurses, chiropractors and other health care professionals
- educators
- beauticians, hairdressers, barbers
- religious leaders
- labor union leaders.

In our Latino community, we determined that religious leaders and folk healers were two of the most influential groups in terms of their ability to influence community members. For this reason, we targeted both these groups for AIDS education.

PAS has worked closely with the Catholic church since the vast majority of Latinos are Catholics. We have been successful in persuading local parish priests to speak from the pulpit encouraging families to talk about HIV/AIDS, urging parents to talk to their children about the subject, and inviting people to participate in our program. Then, as people leave the church services, we hand out AIDS prevention information that has been preapproved by the cooperating clergy. These packets do not contain condoms. However, we explain to those interested where they can obtain them.

In a single Sunday we are able to distribute hundreds of HIV/AIDS prevention kits containing educational materials in both Spanish and English. As we give out the information we tell people the kits contain information they can use to protect their family from AIDS.

This type of outreach has proved effective in opening up dialogue with such groups as sex partners of IDUs, closeted gay and bisexual men, and the family members and friends of those participating in high-risk behavior.

As mentioned above, folk healers are also influential community leaders. In the last three years we have identified and educated four *curanderos* (healers). With this target group, we place special emphasis on providing information on symptoms as well as general AIDS information. We leave educational materials with them and check back on a periodic basis to restock the materials. We are most pleased that this year one of the *curanderos* we had been working with has been recruited for our peer educator training.

Peer Educators

Peer educators are an extremely important part of an outreach program because they are invaluable in overcoming barriers to change. They also foster a sense that community norms are changing which in turn encourages individuals to change.

At PAS we use peer educators to overcome the difficulties inherent in spreading the word about HIV to the Latino community. These obstacles include a cultural tendency not to talk openly about sex; a persistent belief that only gay men can get AIDS; and the fact that many Latino men who have sex with other men do not see themselves as homosexual or bisexual and therefore do not see themselves as engaging in high-risk behavior. These obstacles are best overcome by peer educators who understand intuitively how to get the message across to family, friends, coworkers and neighbors.

Another problem that peer educators easily defuse is that many Latinos, especially those who are undocumented or currently going through the amnesty process, feel either intimidated by or have an animosity toward anyone who appears to be in a position of authority. By their very nature, peer educators are able to defuse such problems.

Media

Mass media—television, radio, magazines, *fotonovelas* and newspapers—can be very powerful enhancers and promoters of your outreach efforts. Make maximum use of them. Although there is a lot of competition in obtaining media coverage, you can with some planning and persistence make the most of the media in your community. Media strategies should be an integral part of your outreach plan.

Making maximum use of the media means assessing which media channels are most popular in your communities. One successful example is the use of radio. We have been very fortunate to have access to KHDC in Salinas. This Spanish language public radio station is the home and work companion to thousands of farmworkers and other Spanish speakers who would otherwise be isolated from the communities they live in. In addition to placing public service announcements, we also participate in the weekly AIDS information program. The use of radio has greatly enhanced our outreach efforts.

Another media channel that is gaining popularity in the United States is the use of *fotonovelas*. *Fotonovelas* are an established mass media channel in Latin America, as popular or more so than newspapers. Latinos, and most especially Mexicans, are accustomed to seeing these being distributed in the United States, and they recognize them as a familiar, popular medium. We have had very positive results in our distribution of AIDS *fotonovelas*. These too have contributed positively to our outreach and educational efforts. Accordingly, you can use the media to heighten the awareness of your community concerning the HIV crisis. Build name recognition for your program, and build both name and visual recognition for your outreach staff, thereby planting the seeds of community trust and acceptance.

Radio, TV and print media can be used to create "a need to know more about HIV prevention" within the community. It is a good idea to use such publicity as a springboard for a large-scale outreach kick-off event. Such an event can be used to blanket the community with basic AIDS information. If successful, it will also serve to foster credibility and increase community acceptance of your program.

Again, public service radio is an important source of low-cost mass media outreach that you can use to the advantage of your HIV education project. Especially in the Spanish-speaking Latino community, where access to information is limited, this type of outreach can be very effective. We have worked closely with the Santa Cruz AIDS Project and KHDC to produce a weekly call-in talk show program entitled "*Una Sola Vida.*" This program allows us to reach thousands of people in our area and provide them with information on the HIV virus on a consistent basis. It also gives our staff more credibility in encountering people who have heard them on the radio because their frequent radio appearances give the CHOWs an air of notoriety, which in turn makes people more interested in their message.

AIDS Awareness Valentine's Day

One successful event was the celebration of AIDS Awareness Valentines' Day to kick off the PAS Latino community street outreach campaign. The Watsonville City Council supported us in this effort by declaring February 14, 1988 as AIDS Awareness Day in the City of Watsonville. This proclamation was extremely valuable to PAS as it gave the event increased credibility and resulted in multi-media news coverage in both Spanish and English.

On the actual day of the event, our volunteers distributed 2,000 AIDS education packets throughout

Watsonville's Main Street and downtown plaza areas. The Latino community was very receptive as evidenced by their interest in the AIDS packets, with many taking time to ask questions about *SIDA* (AIDS). Of the packets handed out, only three were seen thrown on the ground. The rest were observed going into pockets or purses.

This success was due in large part to the discreet way the sexually explicit information (i.e., condom use) was packaged and distributed inside a Valentine's Day card. The PAS volunteers at this event were mostly Latinos—four being monolingual Mexican immigrants, including two women who brought their children, and an older man.

A festive event was made even livelier by having the older children hand out helium-filled balloons to other children, while our adult volunteers distributed sexually explicit HIV/AIDS packets and answered questions. As a result, our AIDS information table in the park, as well as the overall day's events, had a very pronounced Latino flavor.

The success of this event demonstrates that HIV education material (which by its nature requires sexually explicit text and graphics) can be distributed to people in any community if presented in a culturally acceptable manner.

This type of inclusive, intergenerational, community activity works because it can influence community-wide standards and acceptance for AIDS information. This in turn can influence the behavior of individuals within the community.

For AIDS prevention projects to be effective and to produce lasting results they must:

▲ Increase community awareness and knowledge about HIV disease.

▲ Correct commonly held misconceptions about AIDS and reduce community fears.

▲ Create an atmosphere of community support for the adoption of risk-reducing behaviors by individuals at risk for AIDS.

▲ Reduce the rate of HIV transmission/infection by changing the behaviors of at-risk individuals.

A tall order indeed. Since you will never be able to have personal contact with every member or even half of the members of the community, people must be persuaded to pass on AIDS education materials and information to others.

Summary

In developing an outreach strategy suited to the unique needs of your community, remember that no single outreach activity will get the job done. You must combine community involvement and support with a "We can learn from each other" attitude. This, in turn, goes hand in hand with a respect for people's traditions and values. Outreach programs need to be flexible and adaptable to the needs of the community they serve.

Remember that your program must be multifaceted in order to succeed. You should combine street outreach with outreach to your community leaders and a peer educator program if you want to effect behavior change. All these efforts should be accompanied by an ongoing media campaign designed to enhance and promote your outreach efforts.

It is my fond hope that the ideas contained in this chapter will prove useful to you in developing or improving your own AIDS prevention outreach project. Ideally, the information put forth here will serve as a catalyst for the germination of new ideas on how to reach your own community.

13

Evaluating AIDS Education Materials

Shelley Mann, MPH,
and Marna Copeland Taylor, MPH

Introduction

The field of AIDS education has expanded rapidly over the last nine years. Part of that expansion has included the development of educational materials of all types. Central to the design and development of these materials is the often-overlooked process of evaluation.

Evaluation can be done both while a material is being developed (formative evaluation) and after it is completed (outcome evaluation). The purpose of the formative evaluation is to provide information that will enable you to improve the material's effectiveness. It requires input from three different sources: target audience, community members and professionals. While each of these is important, it is the target audience that is the most meaningful. If your audience doesn't understand the information included in your educational material, it is inconsequential whether the community and professionals believe it is effective.

The purpose of the outcome evaluation is to determine how effectively the material meets its educational objectives. Therefore, unless your educational objectives target the community or professionals, only the target audience is studied.

In this section, you will find a discussion of both formative and outcome evaluation methods. By using the suggested evaluation strategies, you can increase the effectiveness of your materials and your knowledge about AIDS education. Since education is such an important tool in preventing AIDS, the knowledge you gain is especially valuable.

Formative Evaluation (Field Testing)

"Field testing" is the term used to describe the process for obtaining the target audience's response to educational materials during the development process. In field tests, representatives of the target audience are asked to evaluate the text, graphics and layout to determine if the material is understandable, relevant, appealing and persuasive. These are the elements which are necessary in order for an educational material to be effective.

The most common methods used to field test are focus groups, individual interviews and written questionnaires. When developing AIDS materials, individual interviews and written questionnaires are most appropriate because sensitive subjects such as contraception and sexual practices are usually discussed. Written questionnaires also guarantee privacy, but they have the disadvantage of requiring higher literacy skills. In addition, written questionnaires do not allow probing. Focus groups are described in detail in Chapter 3, "Using Focus Group Interviews to Design Materials." You can use a combination of focus groups, individual interviews and written questionnaires to gain the advantages each offers.

Written Questionnaires

Advantages:
- answered anonymously
- administered to many people simultaneously
- provide uniform responses because the same information is requested from all respondents

Disadvantages:
- can't probe for more information
- may be hard to persuade people to complete and return them
- impersonal
- require significant literacy skills

Individual Interviews

Advantages:
- flexible so more information can be received
- easier to persuade people to participate
- can explain questions that aren't understood
- can be used with people who have a low level of literacy

Disadvantages:
- time-consuming to administer
- anonymity is not possible
- may produce inconsistent data
- interviewers may influence responses

Each of these methods (as well as focus groups) can be used alone or in combination with each other.

Field testing is not a complicated process, but it can make or break a new material. It provides a crucial opportunity to informally assess your material's potential effectiveness during the development process when changes can easily be made.

Preparation

To begin field testing, produce a mock-up of your material in each language you are producing, including the text and illustrations. The mock-up should be arranged in your proposed format. The copy should be printed or typed, unless you plan to handwrite the final version. Illustrations are important to include, but they don't need to be in final form. This version will change as a result of the field testing, so don't waste your resources on high-quality production.

Next, develop a field test instrument. Since the instrument dictates the quality of the information you will obtain from field testing, plan it carefully. It should have three components: demographics, illustrations, and copy/layout. (See the Instrument Development Guidelines [Figure 13.1] and the Sample Respondent Questionnaire [Figure 13.2].)

Demographics

Only gather demographic information that you will use to determine if you have sampled a cross-section of your target audience or to enable you to analyze your results for different groups. For example, if you are developing an education material for Latino youth, ages 10-15, it is appropriate to ask about age and ethnicity (gender can simply be noted) but maybe not sexual preference or activity.

Figure 13.1

Instrument Development Guidelines

Types of Questions:

▲ *Open-ended:* Respondent is asked to provide his or her own answer. (Example: "What changes would you make after reading this material?")

Advantages:
- flexible
- can document respondents' exact feelings or reactions

Disadvantages:
- hard to score and analyze
- time-consuming

Structure: Fill-in-the-blank; begin with how, when, what, etc.

▲ *Close-ended:* Respondent is asked to select an answer from a specified list given by the interviewer or the questionnaire. (Example: "Would you make any changes after reading this material? Please check all that apply.")

Advantages:
- provides uniform responses
- simple to complete
- easy to score and analyze

Disadvantages:
- not responsive to unique feelings or reactions
- harder to obtain suggestions

Structure: Multiple choice, true/false, yes/no, rating scale

Guidelines for Constructing Questions

▲ Keep questions short and simple. Questions should be able to be read or asked quickly and easily understood.

▲ Make questions clear and precise. Avoid ambiguity in questions so that the person knows exactly what is being asked.

▲ Only ask the information that you need to know.

▲ Use words that your audience will understand.

▲ Begin with the least threatening questions, saving sensitive questions for last.

▲ Provide instructions so respondents know what to do.

▲ **Field test your instrument with a few members of the target audience to make sure that it works.**

Figure 13.2

Sample Respondent Questionnaire
Female Pretest Questionnaire

English/Spanish text   Date _____
                                        Intrvwr _____
age_____ race/ethnic_____   Facility_____
highest grade _____
secur lvl/housing _____

I. Cover
   a. Would you pick up this booklet? Why or why not? _____

   _____

II. Graphics
   a. What is going on in this panel?

Transmission				

   b. What is happening in these pictures?

Myths				
Drugs				
Sex				
Pregnancy				

   c. Do these pictures look like women you know here?_____

   _____

III. Overall
   a. What is the most important thing you learned from this
      brochure? _____

   b. Can you tell me 3 ways to get AIDS?_____

   c. Can you tell me 3 ways to protect yourself from getting
      AIDS?_____

   d. Can you name 4 symptoms of AIDS? _____

e. What are some ways that you can't get AIDS? _____

_____

f. Would you talk to a WAC or IAC person about drug rehab? Why or why not? _____

g. Where would you go to get help if you wanted to get off drugs? _____

h. Can a baby be born with AIDS? How? _____

_____

i. Would you share this booklet with anybody? Who? _____

_____

j. How do you feel after reading this? _____

    ☐ 1. I don't feel any different about AIDS

    ☐ 2. I feel more confused about AIDS

    ☐ 3. I feel I know more about AIDS

    ☐ 4. I feel I am better able to protect myself from AIDS

    ☐ 5. I feel more scared about AIDS

k. What would you change about this booklet? _____

_____

Reprinted with permission from Education Programs Associates, Inc., Campbell, CA. 1988.

Illustrations

We recommend testing illustrations first for comprehension and appeal, before the copy is read. If a person has trouble reading or reads in a language other than the one your material is written in, it is essential that the graphics convey the educational messages. In these situations, the graphics do not just support the text—they speak in place of the text.

Copy/Layout

Your instrument should help you determine the following:

▲   Are the educational messages understandable?

▲   Do the most important points stand out?

▲   Are any aspects of the material offensive?

▲   Is the material considered relevant?

▲   Is the material persuasive, leading to desired changes in knowledge, attitude or behavior?

Preparing for the Field Test

While the instrument is being developed, select your field test group. Be sure to choose people who reflect the characteristics of your target population. It is best if you can test at least 15 clients in each relevant demographic group of concern. If this is not possible, it is far better to obtain some reactions than none at all.

In most cases, the target population will determine the location of the field test. Field testing can be conducted in a variety of places, depending upon the availability of your target audience and the sensitivity of the subject matter. For example, we recently developed a material for parents on discussing AIDS with their teenage children. It was a very short motivational piece which we tested in malls, PTA meetings and flea markets. We have also conducted interviews in people's homes when developing birth control information materials for Southeast Asians. Take precautions to insure the confidentiality and anonymity of field test results to protect the respondents.

Finally, if you plan to conduct focus groups or individual interviews, you need to select and train interviewers. Often the writer of the material will also field test the material. While this is convenient and sometimes the only option, beware of its pitfalls. When the writer conducts field testing interviews, she/he needs to be objective and remain in her/his role as field tester, without getting defensive. Therefore, have at least one other person conduct interviews. A brief training should be conducted for all field testers to discuss the purpose of the process, logistics, questions they may encounter and to review the instrument and material being tested.

Conducting the Field Test

Individual Interviews

At the beginning of each individual interview, be sure to acquaint the respondent with the purpose of your interview. Explain that the material is a draft and you need their assistance to improve it before it is printed. Also inform them of who you are and where you are from. Try to establish a relaxed atmosphere in which the respondent feels safe to offer constructive feedback. Most people are interested in reviewing materials, as long as the process is not lengthy and the material is of interest to them.

During the interview, obtain as much information from each respondent as possible. If a particular section or picture is unclear or misleading, ask for their ideas about how to improve it. More often than not, it is the target audience that has the best ideas about how to explain difficult concepts or depict complex messages. Take advantage of their perspective and ask for help.

If the respondent becomes confused or uncomfortable during the interview, you may need to deviate from the interview instrument. If the respondent finds part of the material confusing, record this information. Don't explain the confusing part of the material at this time, as this is not meant to be an educational session. If education is needed, it should be done after the field test is completed. In addition, if the respondent becomes uncomfortable during the session, it is best to end the interview. Regardless of the results, express your appreciation for the respondent's time and effort.

Written Questionnaires

Written questionnaires are much simpler to administer than individual interviews. The primary challenge of implementing this method of field testing is to insure that the questionnaires are given to the right people and returned to you in a reasonable time period. If someone other than the developers of the material will be distributing the questionnaires (e.g., a clinic receptionist or classroom teacher), it is important to explain the following:

▲ The purpose of the questionnaire

▲ How many questionnaires will be distributed

▲ Who will receive the questionnaire (all or part of a particular group—if a part, whether a random sample the first ten, etc.)

▲ The timeline for completing the questionnaires and returning them

It is advisable to check with the people you have asked to assist you with administering the questionnaires during the field test to make sure that it is proceeding smoothly. If problems have arisen, these can them be solved with minimal disruption to your schedule.

Focus Groups
(See Chapter 3, "Using Focus Group Interviews to Design Materials" for a description of how to conduct focus groups.)

Analyzing the Results

Once you have conducted the interviews or collected questionnaires, it is time to analyze the results. Since you probably are not working with large samples, it can be difficult to generalize. But if two or three of your fifteen respondents find a passage offensive or a particular subgroup finds the pictures misleading, revisions are probably needed. This is when you can use the respondents' ideas for more appropriate wording and graphics.

If interviews were conducted, a post field test meeting of all interviewers is often helpful. The interviewers can give additional insight into respondents' comments and offer their suggestions for improvements. These meetings are especially important if the material is being written in several languages for different cultures. When working on a pamphlet recently, we wanted to incorporate the needs of seven different languages and cultures. During the post field test meeting, the interviewers from each culture brought up changes that should be made to meet their specific cultural/linguistic needs. We discussed how we could incorporate the changes without offending someone else or adding extra pages. It was a long discussion, but some very creative and practical solutions resulted.

When looking at the results, the most critical thing

to assess is whether the key messages were understood. Rewrite the text, reorganize the information, or change the illustrations to eliminate confusion.

The Second Round

After revisions are made, it may be necessary to conduct additional field testing. The purpose of additional tests is to evaluate whether the changes you've made work. This second round of field testing is especially important if major changes were made in the way key messages are presented.

Community Review

When dealing with controversial subjects such as AIDS, it is usually necessary to obtain information about the community's response to the materials you are developing. Field testing with members of the target audience can't tell you about the acceptability of the material to the larger community; it can only tell you about the target audience. For example, with most AIDS materials developed for schools, the broader school community needs to be consulted, even though children or teens are the intended audience. The input of this community—including parents, faculty, administrators and school board—may be essential to insure that the material is sensitive to that community's concerns and will be used.

When deciding whether the larger community needs to review the material, consider the following criteria:

▲ Is anyone's approval necessary before the material can be used?

▲ Could any group or individual block the use of the material?

▲ Is the support of any group or individual crucial to the material's use?

If the answer to any of these questions is "yes," then community members or groups need to review the material. The decision about who should review the material can be difficult. In one case, the specific community groups may be local schools and youth organizations; in another situation, the community of concern may include lesbian and gay organizations and the health department. Refer back to the questions posed in this section to decide whom to include. Just as ignoring an important group can lead to serious problems, asking input from inappropriate groups can also be problematic. Since AIDS can be such a volatile subject, community evaluation can be challenging.

Once you have determined which groups or individuals to involve, clearly state your expectations. In our experiences with community representatives, the evaluation process works best when there are clear ideas about the types of commentary you desire.

The focus of this aspect of the evaluation is to determine whether the material is acceptable. As these people are not the primary target audience, the emphasis is not whether the material is understandable and appealing. The following are sample questions to ask during community evaluations:

▲ How could this material be useful?

▲ Is there anything you think should be changed or added?

▲ Is there anything that you find offensive?

It is essential to tell the community members that they are only one part of the evaluation process and that the target audience and professionals are also re-

179

viewing the material. Let them know how their input will be used and that it will be weighed along with the other information gathered during the evaluation process. This will give them a realistic idea of the process and help reduce the chance of a backlash if all of their input is not incorporated.

The community evaluation can occur in either a group or through individual interviews. We have found groups to be a better gauge at this stage of evaluation unless the approval of key individuals is needed. Groups are also more expedient when several communities need to be considered. They provide a quick sense of the range of opinions within a specific community and frequently can be arranged through established organizations such as community organization boards and PTAs.

If you are developing a series of materials or educational programs, consider establishing a community review board specifically for this purpose. If you are going to establish a new board, be certain to recruit members from all communities who could potentially have an important opinion on the materials to be discussed. Choose people who are aware of their community's needs and can speak to those needs. Participants should also be interested in AIDS education and have the time to devote to the project. Some people may be very knowledgeable and agree to join the board but have other commitments that limit their active participation. If possible, provide board members with "perks," such as free or discounted materials in order to thank them for their contributions or publicly appreciate them in other ways.

Professional Review

Professionals working in the field of AIDS are also important resources during the process of developing materials. In the formative evaluation, there are two different roles for professionals. They are the content experts, whose role is to assess the accuracy and appropriateness of the information and presentation. Professionals are also the gatekeepers, whose acceptance of the material is critical to its dissemination. Both these roles must be incorporated into the professional review.

The most helpful strategy is to be clear about your needs and to set limits on the type of feedback desired. Carefully structure your review process so that you get the information you want and can use.

The following are sample questions to ask professional reviewers:

▲ Are the key messages appropriate for the specified audience?

▲ Is there any information or graphics which are:
  • inaccurate or misleading?
  • unclear or confusing?
  • offensive?

▲ Are there any important points that have been left out?

▲ How would you use the material in your setting?

▲ What audience(s) is it appropriate/not appropriate for?

▲ Does the information contained in this material conflict with any of your settings' policies or processes?

(See Figure 13.3: Sample Professional Review Questionnaire.)

Figure 13.3

Sample Professional Review Questionnaire

Instructions:
Please review the enclosed educational brochure and answer the questions below. Return the completed questionnaire with the material in the enclosed stamped envelope within the next five days. Thank you for your cooperation.

Name_____

Affiliation_____

1. What would you say are the main messages being communicated in this brochure?

2. How important do you think these messages are for young men?
   ____ Very important
   ____ Somewhat important
   ____ Not particularly important

3. In your professional opinion, are the recommendations made regarding condom use appropriate for young men?
   ____Yes ____No   Why?

4. In your opinion, is there any information or graphics in this material that may be offensive or misleading?
   ____Yes ____No   Why?

5. Do you feel that there are any important points relating to this material that may be offensive or misleading?
   ____Yes ____No   Why?

6. Do you feel that there are any important points relating to this topic that have been omitted?
   ____Yes ____No   If yes, what are they?

7. Based on your knowledge of young men, are there any other comments you want to make about this brochure?

THANK YOU FOR YOUR TIME. PLEASE RETURN THIS QUESTIONNAIRE AND THE BROCHURE TO _____
IN THE ENCLOSED ENVELOPE.

Reprinted with permission from Education Program Associates, Inc., Campbell, CA. 1990.

Different professionals frequently have different and even conflicting ideas of how AIDS-related information should be presented. It is helpful to inform reviewers in advance that their comments will be considered along with other evaluation results so that they understand the limitations of their input. Also, remember that you don't need to get everyone's input. Physicians and nurses may need to review some materials, whereas community leaders and activists may be the group to review others.

Professional reviews are usually requested before the material is initially field tested, and then again before it goes to print. The first round guarantees that the information being shown during the field testing is correct, and the second round assures that the changes made after field testing are acceptable.

As with the community reviews, professional evaluation can take place individually or in groups. Groups can provide a setting in which professionals can negotiate solutions to conflicts, simplifying your work as a writer. However, groups have the disadvantage of focusing on dominant members and glossing over the ideas and concerns of less outspoken members. If a group setting is used, try to solicit opinions from everyone present. You can draw on already established professional groups or organize a new group as discussed in the previous section.

Since many of the professionals will play a significant role in distributing your materials, it is essential for them to be involved in the development process. There is a greater chance they will use the material once it is printed if they feel their ideas are integrated into the material.

Remember, professional evaluation is no substitute for testing with the target audience or community review. While professionals provide the bottom line for accuracy, they are not the experts on comprehension, relevance, appeal or community acceptability. The target audience and appropriate community groups are needed to learn about these critical elements. The combined information of these three groups will enable you to make sure that your educational material will best meet your educational objectives.

Outcome Evaluation

After the completion of the field testing, professional reviews and community reviews, the final version of the educational material will be produced. At this stage, the material is ready for use with the target audience and quantitative assessment of how well it meets the educational objectives. Most outcome evaluations consist of a comparison between the target audience's knowledge, attitudes, skills and behavior before and after receiving the material. This assessment is expressed in quantitative terms.

Several caveats need to be addressed here. Since it is rare for an educational material to be used as the sole component of an educational intervention, it is also rare that the outcome of an educational material alone is tested. Educational materials are almost always designed to be part of a health education program, so most outcome evaluations address programs, not materials.

In addition, this type of evaluation can be very expensive, so it may not even be feasible. Finally, if there are no resources to change the material for future printings, it may seem wasteful to the developers. For all these reasons, most people stop their evaluation once the material is reproduced.

In the field of AIDS education, educational materials are such an important tool that they deserve focused attention. It is possible to evaluate the effectiveness of materials, and we urge you to consider budgeting the time and resources for this part of the evaluation process.

Different measures can be used in outcome evaluation, but the most practical ones to assess AIDS-related educational objectives are self-reported. They include the following:

Knowledge

Use multiple choice, fill-in-the-blanks or true/false questions. These questions can be administered in interview or written form, depending on the setting and the literacy of the target audience.

Attitudes

Use Likert scales, a type of measure in which the respondent is presented with a statement and is asked whether they "strongly agree," "agree," "neither agree nor disagree," "disagree" or "strongly disagree." This type of question allows you to find out how strongly a person favors or disfavors a certain attitude or value.

Skills

Use demonstrations to find out if a person has learned a skill from reading your material. Ask them to show you how to do something, e.g., put a condom on a model penis, and rate their performance.

Behaviors

Direct observations or records are the best way to measure behaviors, but with AIDS-related behaviors, these methods are not usually feasible. Instead, you need to rely on self-reports of either behavioral intentions or their current behavior. See Figure 13.4, the Sample Outcome Questionnaire, at the end of this chapter.)

Remember, educational materials are only one part of education. People will not usually change an attitude or behavior by reading a material alone. Behavior and attitude changes are complex and usually result from a multifaceted education program.

Summary

The evaluation process can be an extremely rewarding component of the material development process. Both formative and outcome evaluation can improve all AIDS education efforts, including educational materials.

Often forgotten or minimized, formative evaluations can determine the success of educational materials. Structured feedback from members of the target audience, professionals and relevant community groups will enable you to improve the effectiveness of your materials before they are distributed. A thorough formative evaluation can also provide the data needed to support a large investment into reproduction and dissemination.

Outcome evaluation, while much less common than formative evaluation, focuses on the bottom line—the impact on the target audience. To advance our knowledge of the impact of educational materials on knowledge, attitudes and behavior, we must invest more resources into this type of evaluation.

Both formative and outcome evaluation should play a significant role in all AIDS education efforts, including educational materials. Keep in mind that some evaluation is better than no evaluation. Then use the results to improve your educational efforts and share them with others to improve everyone's knowledge.

Figure 13.4

Sample Outcome Questionnaire
AIDS Questionnaire

AIDS is a very serious health problem in our nation. Health officials are trying to find the best ways to teach people about AIDS. This survey has been developed so you can tell us what you know and how you feel about AIDS. The information you give will be used to develop better AIDS education programs for young people.

DO NOT write your name on this survey. The answers you give will be kept *private*. No one will know what you write. Answer the questions based on what you really know, feel, or do.

Thanks for your help.

PART 1 DIRECTIONS: Read each question carefully, then circle Yes, No, or Unsure in response to the questions below.

Can a person get AIDS from...

1. shaking hands with someone who has AIDS? **Yes   No   Unsure**
2. giving blood? **Yes   No   Unsure**
3. going to school with a student who has AIDS? **Yes   No   Unsure**
4. kissing on the mouth? **Yes   No   Unsure**
5. being bitten by mosquitoes or other insects? **Yes   No   Unsure**
6. sharing needles or syringes used to inject drugs? **Yes   No   Unsure**
7. using public toilets? **Yes   No   Unsure**
8. having sexual intercourse? **Yes   No   Unsure**
9. having a blood test? **Yes   No   Unsure**

Can people reduce their chances of becoming infected with the AIDS virus by...

10. not having sexual intercourse (being abstinent)? **Yes   No   Unsure**

11. using condoms (rubbers) during sexual intercourse? **Yes No Unsure**

12. urinating after sexual intercourse? **Yes No Unsure**

13. having sexual intercourse with only one person who is not infected with the AIDS virus? **Yes No Unsure**

14. not having sexual intercourse with a person who injects or has injected illegal drugs? **Yes No Unsure**

15. taking birth control pills? **Yes No Unsure**

16. Can you protect yourself from becoming infected with the AIDS virus? **Yes No Unsure**

17. Can you tell if a person is infected with the AIDS virus by looking at the person? **Yes No Unsure**

18. Can any person infected with the AIDS virus infect someone else during sexual intercourse? **Yes No Unsure**

19. Can a pregnant woman who has the AIDS virus infect her unborn baby with the virus? **Yes No Unsure**

20. Is there a cure for AIDS? **Yes No Unsure**

21. Are gay men the only people who can get AIDS? **Yes No Unsure**

22. With regard to AIDS, are blood transfusions now generally unsafe? **Yes No Unsure**

23. Do you think you can get AIDS? **Yes No Unsure**

24. Do you know where to get correct information about AIDS? **Yes No Unsure**

25. Do you know where to get tested for the AIDS virus? **Yes No Unsure**

PART 2 DIRECTIONS: Please circle the answer that best describes how you feel about each statement below. Use the following scale:

Agree = I agree with this statement

Disagree = I disagree with this statement

26. Students my age should be taught about AIDS. **Agree Disagree**

27. People should not be afraid of catching AIDS from casual contact, like hugging or shaking hands. **Agree   Disagree**

28. I think that people with AIDS get what they deserve. **Agree   Disagree**

29. The thought of being around someone with AIDS does not bother me. **Agree   Disagree**

30. No one deserves to have a disease like AIDS. **Agree   Disagree**

31. I would not be afraid to take care of a family member with AIDS. **Agree   Disagree**

32. The best way to get rid of AIDS is to get rid of homosexuality. **Agree   Disagree**

33. I would not avoid a friend if he/she had AIDS. **Agree   Disagree**

34. A list of people who have AIDS should be available to everyone. **Agree   Disagree**

35. Students with AIDS have a right to go to my school. **Agree   Disagree**

36. It would not bother me to attend class with someone who has AIDS. **Agree   Disagree**

PART 3 DIRECTIONS: Read each question carefully. Circle the answer that is most appropriate.

37. Have you injected cocaine, heroin, or other illegal drugs into your body? **Yes   No   No Response**

38. Have you shared needles or syringes used to inject drugs? **Yes   No   No Response**

39. Because of AIDS, have you stopped injecting illegal drugs? **Yes   No   No Response**

40. Because of AIDS, have you stopped sharing needles and syringes used to inject drugs? **Yes   No   No Response**

41. Because of AIDS, have ever talked with your boyfriend or girlfriend about AIDS before having sexual intercourse? **Yes   No   No Response**

42. Because of AIDS, have you stopped having sexual intercourse? **Yes   No   No Response**

43. Because of AIDS, have you started using condoms during sexual intercourse? **Yes   No   No Response**

44. Because of AIDS, have you decreased the number of people you have sexual intercourse with? **Yes   No   No Response**

PART 4 DIRECTIONS: Read each statement carefully, then circle the answer that you think is best.

How many persons your age do you think are...

45. having sexual intercourse?
    a. Almost All   b. Most   c. Half   d. Few   e. Almost None

46. using condoms (rubbers) during sexual intercourse?
    a. Almost All   b. Most   c. Half   d. Few   e. Almost None

47. injecting illegal drugs?
    a. Almost All   b. Most   c. Half   d. Few   e. Almost None

48. sharing needles or syringes used to inject drugs?
    a. Almost All   b. Most   c. Half   d. Few   e. Almost None

49. How many people have you had sexual intercourse with *in your life*?
    a. 0   b. 1   c. 2   d. 3 or More   e. No Response

50. How many people have you had sexual intercourse with *in the last year*?
    a. 0   b. 1   c. 2   d. 3 or More   e. No Response

51. How old were you the first time you had sexual intercourse?
    a. 12 or less   b. 13-14   c. 15-16   d. 17-18
    e. Does Not Apply

52. When you have sexual intercourse, how often is a condom used?
    a. Always   b. Sometimes   c. Rarely   d. Never
    e. Does Not Apply

PART 5 DIRECTIONS: Read each question carefully. Circle the correct answer.

53. What grade are you in?
    a. 8th   b. 9th   c.10th   d. 11th   e. 12th

54. What is your sex?
    a. Female   b. Male

55. How old are you?
    a. 12 or Under   b. 13-14   c. 15-16   d. 17-18
    e. 19 Years Old or More

56. What is your race?
    a. White   b. Blsck   c. Hispanic   d. Asian   e. Other

THE END

Thank you for your help. Please return this survey and your answer sheet to the teacher.

AIDS Questionnaire (Answers)

1. No	13. Yes
2. No	14. Yes
3. No	15. No
4. No	16. Yes
5. No	17. No
6. Yes	18. Yes
7. No	19. Yes
8. Yes	20. No
9. No	21. No
10. Yes	22. Yes
11. Yes	23. N/A—Personal Opinion
12. No	24, 25. N/A—Personal knowledge

Reprinted from Quackenbush, M., Nelson, M. and Clark, K., Eds. *The AIDS challenge: Prevention education for young people.* Santa Cruz, CA: Network Publications, 1988.

Appendixes

A

Case Study: Assessing the AIDS Education Needs of Black Gay and Bisexual Men

Stephen B. Thomas, PhD

The subjects (n=91) were adult males, 32 +/- 9 years old, residing in either Baltimore, Maryland or Washington, D.C. who volunteered to answer a confidential survey. The predominant sexual preference reported by the group was gay or homosexual (76.4%), followed by bisexual (20.2%) and heterosexual (2.2%). The majority of the sample were Black (62.7%) and Hispanic (36.1%). Drawn largely from the middle socioeconomic class (50%) and the working class (34.1%), 47.3% reported being employed in professional or managerial positions. Almost 8% were unemployed at the time of the survey. Positive HIV antibodies tests had been received by 15.4% of the group (19.7% of those responding to the question) and 6.7% had been diagnosed with ARC or AIDS.

The subjects reported a range of 0-20 different sexual partners in the month previous to the survey. However, more than half (58%) had one or no partners during this time. Oral sex was the sexual behavior engaged in most frequently by this group. Over one-third of the subjects reported "always" using this form of sexual expression. Anal sex was experienced frequently, but not as often as oral sex; 13.8% indicated "always" and 26.4% "often" engaging in anal sex during a sexual encounter. However, 26.4% reported never having anal sex during the past 12 months.

A low rate of condom use during oral sex practices was revealed. Condoms were never used by 42.7% of the respondents and 14.7% used them "not too often" while participating in this behavior. Over one-half of those sampled used condoms during anal sex (50% "always" and 9.2% "often"). They were "sometimes" or "not too often" used by 22.3%, and "never" used by 18.4% of those responding to the question. Thirty-four subjects reported having vaginal sex with women during the past 12 months. Over one-half (52.9%) of these subjects never used condoms during this activity. Low condom use during oral sex practices and penile-vaginal intercourse was reported. Additionally, almost 20% never used condoms during anal intercourse. Although knowing that having sex with an HIV positive person is risky behavior, one-third of the group indicated having had sex with an HIV positive person, and almost one-fourth said they were likely to practice unsafe sex if they were HIV-positive.

There is a need to further explore attitudes in light of the reported behavior patterns so that interventions may be tailored to reduce the incidence of recidivism. This need is illustrated by looking at parallel attitude and behavior questions. Eighty-percent of the sample disagreed that they would risk getting AIDS for an exciting and wild sexual experience with the right guy. Most of the group felt strongly that it was not "ok" to engage in unsafe sex from time to time and that it was their responsibility to insure safe sex. However, over one-third said that they would be likely to engage in unsafe sex when caught up in the heat of passion. It is suggested that role plays addressing certain specific interpersonal situations be incorporated into AIDS education targeted to this population.

Source: Thomas, S. and G. Hodges. 1989. Assessing the AIDS needs of Black men who have sex with other men: A pilot study. Technical Report submitted to National Association of Black and White Men Together, Los Angeles, CA.

B

Case Study: Stopping AIDS Is My Mission (SAMM)

Aisha Gilliam, EdD

Stopping AIDS Is My Mission (Thomas, 1988) is an AIDS prevention and education project whose primary objectives are to:

▲ Organize the SAMM Coalition and mobilize the community.

▲ Assess the AIDS education needs of the target community.

▲ Assess the efficacy of selected AIDS messengers.

▲ Develop culturally appropriate AIDS education materials.

This case study describes the process of evaluating AIDS educational materials, reflecting the fourth point above. A total of 48 community-based organizations (CBOs), federal agencies, state and local governmental agencies and national organizations were selected from the February 1988 edition of the Local Directory of AIDS Related Services, published by the U.S. Conference of Mayors (USCM). Organizations funded to provide AIDS education for minority populations were identified by a USCM official. A letter of request was sent, followed by a second letter one month later if no information was received.

Items received from responding agencies or organizations were labeled with an identification number to indicate the type of print medium and the year of publication. A four-digit number was assigned to each document to facilitate retrieval from the Minority Health Research Laboratory computer database of AIDS educational materials. For example, the code 86-0001-BR refers to brochure (BR) number 001, published in 1986. Where the actual year of the publication was not available, the year in which it was received by the MHRL was used. Because of the ongoing research in AIDS, the staff saw a need to recognize when a certain publication was made available to the target audience.

Information received by SAMM included brochures, booklets, pamphlets, reports, newsletters, information cards, information brochures describing the responding organizations, posters and other miscellaneous items labeled "Other," (e.g., sample condom packets and a pocket sized guide for proper needle cleaning).

Overall, materials received were coded according to the primary target audience, i.e., designed for the general public, health professionals, American Indians, Chinese Americans, Latinos and/or Black Americans, intravenous drug users, women, teens, gay/lesbian men and women, business professionals, hemophiliacs, or criminal justice professionals. Figure B.1 represents the coding of the first 32 items received by SAMM, Glenarden Project. Figure B.2 represents the document coding key (*Webster's Ninth New Collegiate Dictionary*, 1987).

Most of the organizations that responded were those providing answers to requests for information from people concerned about or affected by AIDS and HIV infection. There was a low response rate from or-

Figure B.1

Selected AIDS Education Materials for Minority Populations (SAMM)

CODE	TITLE	TG	SRC	RDG	GEN CHAR
1. 88-0001-IB	BEBASHI, Blacks educating Blacks about sexual health issues	BK	8	16	GR
2. 88-0002-BR	AIDS IN THE BLACK COMMUNITY: THE FACTS	BK	8 47	10	GR PR
3. 88-0003-BR	YOU DON'T HAVE TO BE WHITE OR GAY TO GET AIDS	ALL	8 44	7	GR PR CO
4. 88-0004-BR	WHAT YOU SHOULD KNOW ABOUT AIDS	GP	11	10	GR
5. 88-0005-BR	PELIGRO GRAVE: AIDS/SIDA Y LAS DROGAS	LA	3		SP CO
6. 88-0006-BR	AIDS/SIDA Y EL SEXO SEGURO	LA	3		CO SP
7. 88-0007-BR	¡PROTEJASE CONTRA AIDS/SIDA! - TAMBIEN ES UN PROBLEMA	LA	3		SP CO
8. 88-0008-BR	AIDS AND SAFER SEX	GP	3		AS CO
9. 88-0009-BR	SOME STRAIGHT ANSWERS ABOUT AIDS AND IV DRUGS	IV	3	10	CO
10. 88-0010-BR	AIDS - IT'S A BLACK PROBLEM, TOO	BK	3	10	CO
11. 87-0011-IC	WOMEN, INFANTS AND AIDS	WO	20	10	AS
12. 87-0012-IC	MUJERES, INFANTES Y "AIDS" (SIDA)	LA WO	20	6	SP
13. 87-0013-BR	YOU DON'T HAVE TO BE WHITE OR GAY TO GET AIDS	BK	20	6	GR CO
14. 87-0014-BR	ANDREA AND LISA	TN	20	7	GR CO
15. 88-0015-BR	REACH FOR THE BLEACH	IV	20	8	GR CO
16. 88-0016-CA	HERO CATALOG	HP GP	20	A	GR CO
17. 87-0017-BR	WOMEN AND AIDS	WO	18 44	10	GR CO
18. 87-0018-BR	LAS MUJERES Y EL SIDA	LA WO	18 44	11	PR GR CO AS
19. 87-0019-BR	SOBRE EL SIDA Y EL INYECTARSE DROGAS	LA IV	18		GR SP PR CO
20. 87-0020-BR	ABOUT AIDS AND SHOOTING DRUGS	IV	18	11	GR SP PR CO
21. 86-0021-BR	COPING WITH AIDS	HP	18		GR AS PR CO
22. 86-0022-BR	ALCOHOL, DRUGS & AIDS	IV	18 44	11	PR
23. 86-0023-BR	ALCOHOL, DROGAS Y AIDS	IV	18	11	GR AS PR CO
24. 86-0024-BR	AIDS/SIDA: ¡INFORMESE!	LA	18	11	GR SP PR CO
25. 88-0025-BR	SEXUAL HEALTH REPORTS, SPRING 88, VOLUME 9:1	GL	31		SP PR CO

Figure B.2

Document Coding Key

SAMPLE:

| 8 | 6 | — | 0 | 0 | 0 | 1 | — | B | R |

yr of publication   item number   type of medium

BROCHURE	**BR**	contains advertising or descriptive materials; pamphlet; booklet
PAMPHLET	**PM**	an unbound printed publication with no cover or with a paper cover
BOOKLET	**BK**	a little book; especially, pamphlet
POSTER	**PO**	a bill or placard for posting often in a public place; specifically, one that is decorative or pictorial
OTHER	**O**	condom packets, etc.
INFO CARD	**IC**	contain basic information about AIDS
REPORT	**RE**	a written record or summary of study in some AIDS-related topic
INFO BROCHURE	**IB**	describes organizational source of document
CATALOGUE	**CA**	contains items available for distribution from groups that produce and sell AIDS-related educational materials
NEWSLETTER	**NE**	a printed sheet, pamphlet, or small newspaper containing news or information of interest chiefly to a special group

Definitions from: *Webster's Ninth New Collegiate Dictionary,* (1987). Springfield, MA: Merriam-Webster Inc.

ganizations providing direct services. Organizations providing education responded with the most culturally appropriate materials available at the time of the request.

Determining Reading Levels of Items

Freimuth (1979) reports that there are least 40 readability formulas available for predicting the grade level at which a reader can understand a specific message. Of these, the SMOG Grading Formula developed by McLaughlin (1979) was used to determine the readability levels of selected items received by the SAMM, Glenarden (Maryland) project. A convenience sample of items targeted for Black audiences was selected from the domain of all materials received. Fifty-nine percent had reading levels of 8th grade or lower, while 41% of the items ranged from reading levels of grades 10 to 16.

First, staff reaction to the materials was obtained. The materials considered most appropriate were then chosen to be presented for review by residents. Central location intercept interviews were carried out in malls and on location in the housing complex to determine the acceptability, comprehension and relevance of the various pamphlets. A guide was used by the trained staff person conducting the interviews. Items that were difficult to comprehend and those that created confusion were deleted from the selection of sample items made available to this population.

Developing Materials

The focus group results were used along with the MHRL AIDS Prevention Survey to obtain information about the dynamic relationships of attitudes, opinions

and behaviors on a wide range of issues relating to AIDS. Specifically, the focus groups on this project were designed to obtain information about and insight into the following areas:
- knowledge, attitudes and beliefs (KAB)
- prevention of infection
- drug use
- sexuality
- treatment of People with AIDS (PWAs)
- community resources
- prevention and Education to reach minorities

Key Factors Identified

A great deal of information was made available as a result of the focus group and the AIDS prevention survey. The survey results provided insight into information deficits, while focus groups elicited information about why people felt the way they did, reasons for their behaviors and the contextual framework for conduct of behavior. The following are comments derived from the focus groups' study considered important in designing the first two brochures.

"I don't believe that Black people get AIDS any more than White people—lies, lies, lies."

"Those places, CDC, the Health Department, they lie about hypertension—they'll lie about AIDS."

"They just want Black people to feel inferior, like we're the only ones that get diseases."

"Anything that's bad comes from our community or Africa—that's what they'll like us to believe."

"We don't mind being around them (PWAs), but we don't want our children exposed to those kind of people."

"Children are innocent, they're our future."

"Our own kind should spread the word—people we can trust, like Jesse Jackson. Then they might listen."

"AIDS makes me afraid because I don't want to suffer. We all die, but I'm scared of suffering."

Procedures

The purpose was to develop an educational pamphlet which would:

- communicate the seriousness of AIDS in the Black community
- grasp the attention of those reading the pamphlet
- include motivators for action
- present information about what can be done to prevent the spread of AIDS.

In designing the first draft of the brochure, many of the issues addressed in the focus groups were taken into consideration. These represented areas of misinformation which included the severity of the disease, belief in casual contact, the threat to personhood, roots to historical past, the importance of children in the community, and distrust of the establishment. The following steps were therefore taken in order to produce an effective product appropriate for the target audience:

1 Specify the target group.

2 Identify the availability and appropriateness of existing materials.

3 Determine the appropriate media channels for reaching the target audience.

4 Select or develop the materials best suited for the message to:

- provide factual information;
- provide skills to improve efficacy of behavior change;
- provide motivators for risk reduction.

5   Define intended outcomes.

Specifying the Target Group

The brochure to be developed was aimed at residents at the Glenarden housing project. Residents were Black adults and their children, reflecting households with an average income of $10,000, and an average educational level of 9th grade. Characteristics that place this group at risk include drug use and sexual activity.

Appropriate Materials and Media Likely to Reach the Group

Postcards addressed to residents and sent through the mail were identified by the residents in the focus groups as one way to catch the attention of adults in the households. Flyers placed under the door or handed out were cited as less effective.

Facts to Be Included in the Message

Outreach workers (who were also members of the community) felt that it was important to let people know that Blacks were also at risk for AIDS, and that they got AIDS in disproportionate numbers. They also felt that information should be included on ways to prevent AIDS and the message that children can get AIDS from their mothers. The address or location of the SAMM project office and the telephone number were also included in case individuals wanted more information or a referral.

Motivators for Preventing or Changing Risk Behavior

Several potential themes were considered for the brochure. A theme of "Dreams" based on the famous speech by Dr. Martin Luther King (MLK) was selected because of its widespread familiarity in the Black community and the positive light in which he is held as a role model. This was reinforced by the insertion of a poem by Langston Hughes that emphasized idioms of the black language patterns to draw upon MLK's idea of a dream in the language of the audience. The notions of freedom and a future for the children were suggested as important ideas in motivating adults to take action on behalf of their innocent children whom they hold dear. These examples represent long-term consequences that hold potential for initiating change in the target population.

Improved efficacy skills are of the utmost importance in preventing or changing behavior. For this reason, a method of preventive behavior was included on all brochures produced. To improve their skills, community residents may need greater intervention, since prevention actions include:

▲ Interpersonal skills (e.g., negotiating, decision making, self-management)

▲ Practical skills (e.g., using condoms, practicing safe sex techniques).

Therefore, in addition to information about the location of the office, flyers are distributed weekly to announce to workshops offered to teach these skills. Individuals also receive workshop information if they call. This convenient contact within the community provides an avenue for social support offered by staff, and through participation in the many weekly skills and peer groups, serves as a built-in motivator for behavior change.

205

Intended Outcomes

These are two-fold: keeping hope alive, and achieving the general reduction of AIDS in the community. Breaking the chain of disease and death is likened to that of slavery, a concept which most Blacks well understand. This negative consequence through imagery is part of the message and is designed to trigger a low level of anxiety to reduce further denial within this population. To accomplish this, preventive behaviors are emphasized in the brochure.

Pretesting Brochures

The initial draft was distributed to a selected group of professionals for assessment of relevance, clarity, appropriateness and correctness of factual information. In addition, a focus group discussion of 10 residents ranging in ages from 13 to 45 was convened. The brochure was also pretested with a group of gatekeepers—health professionals acting as intermediaries to review and/or approve materials—and Black professional staff.

Feedback from Black Professionals

The feedback from Black professionals was more critical of the materials than the feedback from the target audience. Here are some of the comments received:

"Instead of enclosing several facts, only one fact at a time should be included for this population."

"Bare essentials should be included, since those who may not read all of the words will still get the gist of the message."

"The brochure is too technical."

"Presentation of statistics may frighten individuals into no action."

Figure B.3

Focus Group Interview

**Focus Group Interview Guide
for AIDS Education Materials for SAMM Project**

Target Audience _____
# of Respondents _____
Location _____
Moderator _____
Observer(s) _____
Interview Date _____

1. What idea is this card (brochure) trying to get across to you?
2. Does it tell you to do anything?
3. How do you feel about the statistics (numbers) presented?
4. Is there anything about this card that might be offensive?
5. Is there anything about this card that is confusing to you?
6. Is there anything you like about this card?
7. Is there anything you dislike about this card?
8. Do you think people in your community will read it?
9. Do you think the people in your community will understand it?
10. Describe in general how you feel about this brochure.

"The brochure is too busy; people may not get the idea."

"There is nothing about AIDS on the front of the brochure and this may be misleading."

"Inclusion of chains may reinforce the idea that Whites are spreading the disease.

Feedback from Gatekeepers:

"The reference to Dr. Martin Luther King is very positive."

207

"People will be curious to open the card when they see a picture of Dr. King, but if you put AIDS on it they may throw it out."

"Breaking the chain may make people take this seriously since they might see the threat to the Black race as a whole."

"The emphasis on children is positive since some residents who don't care much about their own bodies may yet take action on behalf of their children."

"There may be a few too many facts in the brochure, making it seem overwhelming."

"The print size of the words should be made larger, and fewer words should be included." "Several different cards can be made emphasizing a variety of facts so the focus can zero in on one thing at a time."

Focus Group Discussion
with Members of the Target Audience

Individuals were able to identify the main idea of the brochure, that of stopping AIDS in the community. Everyone was able to cite ways to prevent the spread and actions they should take mentioned in the brochure. Nothing about this brochure was cited as offensive; on the contrary, the audience made many positive comments about the card. Although individuals felt that the brochure was easy to understand, some of the younger individuals felt that the incidence of AIDS among the women was unbelievable. In addition, a few children (age 13) misinterpreted the meaning of some of the statistics.

The fact that Dr. King was on the front of the card was the most popular feature of the brochure. Many felt that he was a positive focus in the community, and many said they would look at the brochure and keep it around for a while. They felt that other pamphlets get thrown into the garbage immediately; however, if each family receives one personally addressed to them, they will read it and share the information. People liked the poetry and the emphasis on saving the children. The children stressed the bright look on the face of the child in the brochure. The adults related the chains in the picture to the drug usage and violence in the community. All indicated that they liked the card, and they felt it was believable—especially because it came from SAMM, with which they are familiar. The card along with the group educational activities were acknowledged as effective ways of providing AIDS education in their community as it addressed all Black people.

Revision of Cards

The cards were revised to take into account some of the suggestions made by both groups. Several cards were designed to accommodate a particular risk factor and appropriate behaviors to reduce that risk factor. An example of one card is included in Figures B.4-5. By developing different cards for different risk factors, SAMM designers could avoid overwhelming individuals with too many facts, as suggested by professionals and gate-keepers. It was also deemed important to design a card especially for the children in the community, citing ways they too could help stop the spread of AIDS. Since many parents sent their children to the slide shows offered by SAMM, these children now show great interest in learning about AIDS. An additional motivator, "a magic number," was included. The idea was to increase the likelihood that people will keep and read the card with the hope of winning a prize.

Dissemination of Cards

Cards were addressed and sent to the primary adult in each household based on the resident list from the SAMM management office. On the back of each card was a number, representing a lottery pick. Each month a number is drawn, and that household receives a prize donated by one of the businesses in the community. This procedure is designed to ensure that households keep their cards. Each month a new card is disseminated with different facts and accompanying risk reduction behaviors. Motivators for action will be different but the emphasis will be on an Afrocentric approach.

Assessing Effectiveness

The SAMM office keeps a computerized mailing list of residents. As the cards are distributed, information is kept on the date of distribution, the type of card and the "magic number." Follow-up calls are made to a sample of residents by outreach workers. Questions are asked, similar to those in the focus group discussion. Those residents without phones are reached door to door, and a similar interview conducted. This process is repeated on a monthly basis, with a record kept of those who were interviewed. These contacts also serve to inform individuals of other educational events being offered by the SAMM program in the community. Information obtained is then fed back to the SAMM program.

Summary

The process of developing AIDS educational materials for a particular community requires collaborative efforts. Through a series of actions—defining the target group, assessing its needs, matching messages to materials and

Figure B.4

SAMM Card Side 1

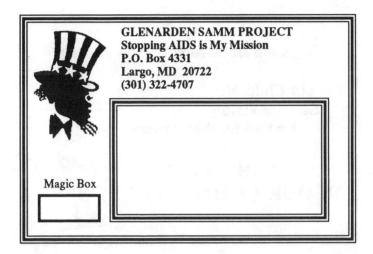

GLENARDEN SAMM PROJECT
Stopping AIDS is My Mission
P.O. Box 4331
Largo, MD 20722
(301) 322-4707

Magic Box

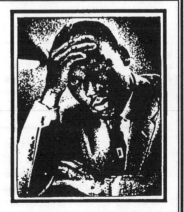

Don't Let
This
  Man's
    DREAM
Become a
  *"Dream
  Lost."*

Figure B.5

SAMM Card Side 2

Keep Hope Alive!

Let our Children
See the Vision
he had for their Future!

**FIGHT AIDS
IN OUR COMMUNITY !**

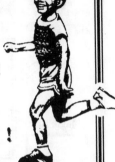

52% OF ALL CHILDREN WITH AIDS ARE BLACK

These children do not have AIDS because
they are Black, they have AIDS because:
- Their mothers shoot drugs
- Their mothers' sex partners shoot drugs

Knowledge Can Protect You!
GET THE FACTS! CALL:
- 1-800-342-AIDS (The National AIDS Hotline)
- 1-(301) 322-4707 (Stopping Aids is My Mission Project Office)
  (8435 Hamlin Street, Apt. #201)

media channels, and testing material effectiveness (readability and response levels)—educators can coordinate AIDS educational campaigns that are culturally appropriate for a given target group.

AIDS education programs can incorporate a variety of ways to promote efficacy skills. In this case study, for example, workshops to improve interpersonal and practical skills were made available to the target community.

Finally, educators must learn to choose culturally-sensitive facts and formats to reach their audience most effectively. In this way, intended outcomes can be both defined and achieved.

References

Freimuth, V.S. 1979. Assessing the readability of health education messages. *Public Health Reports* 94(6): 568-70.

Thomas, B. (Principal Investigator.) Stopping AIDS is My Mission (SAMM): A community coalition model for AIDS education prevention and risk reduction in the Black community. Robert Wood Johnson Grant no. 14629.

C

Case Study: Conducting Outreach to Combat AIDS Among Injection Drug Users*

Robert S. Broadhead, PhD,
and Kathryn J. Fox, MA

Introduction

Injection drug users (IDUs) represent the second largest group at risk for spreading and contracting HIV, and many outreach projects, some funded by the National Institute on Drug Abuse, are presently working with this population and their sexual partners to curb the epidemic. Central to outreach projects are "Community Health Outreach Workers," or CHOWs as they are sometimes called. CHOWs attempt to work directly with IDUs on their own terms and turf and teach them about the risk of AIDS and how they can protect themselves and others.

In "taking the project to the streets," CHOWs confront several problems of work that are virtually identical to the central methodological problems social scientists face in conducting ethnography or field research.

*This research is funded by the National Institute on Drug Abuse (DA-05517) This document was a poster presentation at the Fifth International Conference on AIDS in Montreal, Canada, June 4-9, 1989 by Robert S. Broadhead, PhD, University of Connecticut, and Kathryn J. Fox, University of California, Berkeley.

Among these problems are:

▲ Establishing a very unusual but credible identity within communities that harbor distrust of others, especially outsiders;

▲ Socially mapping and analyzing communities in order to understand them "from the points of view of community members";

▲ Forming relationships with IDUs, prostitutes, and others, yet controlling the level and impact of one's participation;

▲ Cultivating and sustaining a viable role in the field.

Methods

This is an ongoing ethnographic study of the dynamics of outreach work conducted in a demonstration outreach project in a major city on the West Coast. At present the project consists of 22 CHOWs divided equally in number between men and women. Ethnically, there are ten African-Americans, seven Hispanics, four Whites and one Asian. The CHOWs are organized into six teams working in different targeted areas of the city that have been found, via ethnographic and epidemiological methods, to contain large numbers of IDUs and others at risk of AIDS.

The authors have been in the field as participant observers for a year and will continue for another fifteen months. We have also been conducting extensive formal interviews with Project staff members. Broadhead divides his time attending key administrative meetings involving the project directors, supervisors and the CHOWs, and on the street both observing CHOWs in action and working as a CHOW with a three-member team deployed in a large Latino community. Fox works similarly with a six-member team in the city's large sex trade zone, and with a three-member team assigned to an area that contains large numbers of homeless and runaway youth. A former field researcher with our project, Gayle Williams, also spent over six months with a CHOW team working primarily with the female sexual partners of IDUs.

In order to maximize our participation as members of outreach teams, and to investigate the lived experience of being CHOWs, the authors completed the Project's two-week outreach training program. The training also certified us, which helped overcome some of the distrust that many CHOWs held toward us in wanting to observe them in action, or working as CHOWs ourselves alongside them. One one hand, many CHOWs suspected that we would be evaluating their performance and reporting back to their supervisors; it took us a long time to assure them otherwise.

On the other hand, our backgrounds are very different from most of the CHOWs. For example, although we were allowed to train as outreach workers along with newly hired recruits, it is very unlikely that the project would have actually hired either of us had we applied for the job, primarily due to our lack of "real world" street experience. In contrast, while some of the CHOWs have considerable formal education and training, and others have impressive trade skills and job histories, most were hired because their backgrounds reflected a special combination of conventional and street-based credentials. Indeed, there is a collective pride among those CHOWs who have converted a painful and stigmatizing experience, such as drug or alcohol addictions or a prison record, into an asset that prepares them to work on the street with populations at risk of contracting AIDS.

Establishing an Identity

Entering into communities and working with members on their own terms is a problematic endeavor, even with previous street savvy and experience. Because CHOWs interact with people who use illicit drugs and may also engage in other illegal activities, they must first convince community members that they are not narcs or another kind of undercover agent. Suspicion and paranoia toward strangers run high in communities that are most at risk of AIDS, and especially toward individuals who "do not mind their own business." Also, community residents have their own turf and street-based reputations to protect. They can become suspicious when apparent outsiders move into home territories and begin making claims about helping people to save themselves. Thus, in beginning outreach work, all CHOWs face a methodological problem central to ethnography itself: establishing an *identity* of who they are and what they do, that they can be trusted, and that they work to understand and help a community from the point of view of its members.

Initially, CHOWs establish their reputations by distributing condoms and small bottles of bleach to IDUs and others as they walk the streets. The symbolic as well as practical significance of these gifts is enormous. Foremost, in realizing that the gifts can protect them from a deadly incurable disease, community members cannot help but feel good about CHOWs and their work in the community. Symbolically, the gesture of placing small bottles of bleach or condoms in IDUs' hands conveys, in a most dramatic way, that CHOWs are in their communities to help them in a nonjudgmental way. CHOWs become quickly associated with the bleach and condoms they distribute. On occasion, they fill bleach bottles publicly, or set up tables on the streets with plenty of bleach, condoms and literature, making themselves available for clients. These public displays strengthen CHOWs' primary identities as health workers.

There are several other methods CHOWs use to establish their identities on the streets. For example, CHOWs who are new to a community can benefit from the credentials of an established CHOW introducing and vouching for them. CHOWs also enlist the help of clients they do not know to *sponsor* them, as one explained:

> "When I first started working the streets and I met someone who was 'in the mix,' I'd asked him to walk with me: 'Come on, help me hand this stuff out.' Thus clients helped me become known."

Finally, CHOWs establish their identities by staying in *constant contact* with their communities and their known clients. Effective outreach cannot be part-time or erratic work. A CHOW's presence, as it confirms his or her identity, must be consistent. Also, because client populations tend to be transient, and therefore everchanging, CHOWs must work to sustain continuity.

Cultural Analysis and Social Mapping

To understand and help a community from the point of view of its members, CHOWs must empirically study a community as ethnographers do through systematic, personal involvement. They work to identify the cultural and religious backgrounds of community members, their class and ethnic composition, the different languages and dialects spoken, rules of etiquette, community customs and rituals, and attitudes toward work, family, marriage, politics, health and illness, and, of course, drugs.

CHOWs also work to understand the geography of clients' communities: their neighborhoods, hangouts, meeting places, territorial boundaries, housing projects, hotels, bars, community agencies, and the daily or weekly schedules that members follow in frequenting different areas.

Finally, CHOWs attempt to map the social organization of community members: their local and street-based hierarchies, the location of opinion-leaders, gangs, and competing groups, and the different status systems that community members use to rank one another. For example, as one of the project directors emphasized:

> "If someone has a heavy reputation on the street, remember, it was *achieved*. People have careers on the street, and you have to understand the terms in which that respect was earned."

CHOWs' reliance on the information they obtain from opinion leaders is similar to ethnographers' dependence upon key informants and gatekeepers.

Conducting Participant Observation

Based on their ethnographic reading of communities, CHOWs begin the delicate task of approaching IDUs and others on the street. Observational data indicate that CHOWs fashion very different styles of approaching and interacting with community members, but that each one's style emerges somewhat out of trial and error. As one CHOW described:

> "Early on, I tried walking up to people and asking them if they wanted some bleach, but I got some really strong reactions to that. It can really offend people. So I've had to re-examine my style."

With experience, CHOWS become adept at identifying

and approaching the right people, and in ways that avoid problems. The most important characteristic of successful methods of approaching clients is that of *discretion:* CHOWs' interactions must be sensitive and sufficiently private to assure clients' confidentiality. Put another way, the greater the public exposure and visibility of CHOW-client interactions, or the number of "eyes that see it," the more difficult the interaction. Public exposure increases the clients' risk of being identified as drug users, prostitutes, or others in precarious circumstances. A low profile and circumscribed style reduces clients' risk of exposure. In accompanying CHOWs in the field, we have commented that people frequently appear defensive and nervous in accepting the bleach. "That's why," as one CHOW explained, "I just hold it in my hand and pass it to them—just like it was a drug deal." Another CHOW, working in a Latino area, used a street expression to describe bleach transactions: *bajo el ala* or *la mesa* ("under the wing" or "table").

Generally, as the criminal risks of drug use and levels of surveillance by narcotics squads increase, IDUs are driven further underground, which means that CHOWs must be even more discreet in accessing and working with them. Ironically, however, as CHOWs' reputations grow and they become more outstanding in the community, the greater is the likelihood that clients can be seen interacting with them, and the more that others can read into those interactions. Thus, in conducting effective outreach, CHOWs must work to establish widely their community reputation; but, in actually contacting clients, they must work in discreet ways on the street in order to minimize client's risk of public exposure. The need to be discreet explains why CHOWs frequently pass bleach bottles to IDUs in a furtive, clandestine manner that can resemble a drug transaction.

They also reduce public visibility of their activities by dressing down: most CHOWs do not wear conspicuous clothing or insignia that identify them as outreach workers. As one CHOW explained with a smile: "We don't wear badges out here."

Creating A Viable Role

CHOWs must balance the amount of time and effort they invest in helping individual clients *versus* distributing AIDS-prevention materials widely throughout their assigned community.

To establish their reputation, CHOWs work to help individuals deal with a wide assortment of problems. But, in working with individuals, CHOWs can become quickly inundated with the enormity and complexity of clients' problems. CHOWs' primary clients live in extraordinarily deprived circumstances.

Additionally, once IDUs realize that CHOWs can be trusted and want to work with people on their own terms, they exhibit tremendous dependency and make enormous demands: help in finding shelter, food, transportation, medical care, child care, admission to drug treatment, application for government assistance, money, cigarettes, and of course, condoms and bleach. The level of expressed need can be simply overwhelming. But, in working on individual cases, CHOWs' distribution of AIDS prevention materials in the field can become significantly displaced.

In addition, CHOWS can come to experience feelings of powerlessness in trying to help many clients; the interplay of drugs, poverty, AIDS, and death, combined with the lack of real alternatives or resources that can be brought to bear, can be enormously frustrating day after day. The personal costs and risks to CHOWs' own health and well being in conducting outreach have yet to be fully understood.

Conclusion

The methodological problems that CHOWs face in conducting outreach parallel many of those in doing ethnography, although they must be solved in different ways. Much of the literature on ethnography focuses on the problem of how researchers cultivate a place for themselves in situations in which they have no natural role or membership—they are outsiders. But the Project, like most other outreach projects in the country to our knowledge, hires people who are indigenous to the communities in which they work.

As ethnographers, CHOWs face the dual problems of having to cultivate an unusual role for themselves, and gain some perspective on the indigenous membership roles that they already have. CHOWs recognize that they are hired in large part for their community membership, yet some CHOWs fail to realize that they need to create a new role for themselves. Thus, CHOWs obviously need substantial ethnographic training in knowing what their work is about, and how to solve the methodological problems they face in the field. Projects which simply assume that, because CHOWs are indigenous they already know how to make their way in the community, are setting themselves up for major disappointment in staff performance. Just like ethnographers, CHOWs need to learn how to make their way in the community in a substantially new way.

Contributors

Robert S. Broadhead, PhD, is an associate professor of sociology at the University of Connecticut. His current studies focus on the societal responses to AIDS and drug users. Dr. Broadhead works in the field as a participant observer and is conducting extensive, formal interviews with CHOW Project staff. In addition to his work as a field observer, he works as a CHOW with a three-member team in a large Latino community.

Dominic Cappello works as an independent art director and producer, developing print and audio-visual materials for education. His most recent projects include: *The California Wellness Guide* for the State Department of Mental Health; *Consider the Connections,* a video on drug use and sexual decision making for the University of California at Berkeley; Bleachman's *Use A Condom* bus shelter poster for the San Francisco AIDS Foundation; prototype video programs for the Northwest Regional Educational Laboratory's California Pedagogy Project; and *Seasons,* The National Native American AIDS Prevention Center's quarterly. Cappello is also president of the board of directors of Human Health Organization and art director of *OUT/LOOK Magazine*. He is currently working on a fully illustrated guide to HIV care.

Lianne B. Chong is the managing partner and senior art director of L. Chong Designs Associates, a visual communications firm based in San Francisco, California. Ms. Chong has over seventeen years of professional experience in her field. Since 1985, she has helped non-profit organizations in various Pacific Asian communities develop printed materials for health and educational issues. Ms. Chong has also assisted agencies in instituting identity programs for social service projects. She is currently working with profit sector companies and corporations in creating multilingual, culturally sensitive visual materials.

Joyce V. Fetro, PhD, is the health education curriculum specialist for the San Francisco Unified School District. Dr. Fetro received a master's degree in school health education with a primary focus on research instrument development and her doctoral degree from Southern Illinois University in community health education with a special emphasis in educational research and evaluation. Dr. Fetro has extensive experience in qualitative and quantitative research methodology and statistics, as well as experience in applied research and instrument development. She has developed instruments to measure knowledge, attitudes and behaviors in various health-related areas and has conducted content analyses. She is also experienced in conducting focus group interviews and in the development of needs assessments.

Kathryn J. Fox, MA, is an advanced graduate student at the University of California at Berkeley whose doctoral dissertation will be in the areas of drug policy and social deviance.

Sarah Olivia Garcia is the associate director for the Center for Equity and Cultural Diversity at Educational Development Center, Inc. (EDC) in Newton, MA. She is a certificated educator with extensive experience in training on multicultural issues and populations. She currently coordinates a Community AIDS Prevention Project for Inner City Hispanic Youth and a Women at High Risk AIDS Prevention Project, involving development of site-specific materials in Spanish and English for locations in Puerto Rico, Mexico and Connecticut. Her experience includes serving as a master trainer for the Curriculum on Cultural Approach to the Prevention of HIV Infection Among Hispanic Women, as well as providing cultural diversity training for colleges and organizations throughout the eastern and southwestern United States.

Aisha Gilliam, EdD, is an assistant professor and health coordinator of the health education program at Howard University, Washington, DC. She holds a doctorate from Columbia University. Dr. Gilliam's background is in health and human behavior. She has worked extensively in the community, designing and evaluating health programs. She is presently involved in qualitative analysis of community-based AIDS education programs.

Andrea Green Rush is the director of information services for the National Native American AIDS Prevention Center (NNAAPC) in Oakland. She is the editor of *Seasons*, the Center's quarterly newsletter and compiles the Center's Resource Catalog. She also coordinates a number of the agency's information services including its clearinghouse and hotline. Prior to working at NNAAPC she worked for the Institute of Transportation Studies Library in the University of California at Berkeley and has published several biographies on transportation-related subjects. Ms. Green Rush was born and raised in Los Angeles, California and is of Black, Hispanic and Miskito Indian descent.

Roberta Hollander, PhD, is an associate professor in health education at Howard University, Washington, DC. She holds a doctorate in sociology from American University, Washington, DC. She also earned a masters of public health from Johns Hopkins University in Baltimore, MD, and was a post-doctoral fellow there in behavioral sciences-health education. Dr. Hollander has carried out research and published widely on work and health issues, especially with respect to women. Her recent work includes AIDS in the workplace, and women and AIDS.

Susan A. Leibtag, MLS, is librarian of the Media/Materials Center at the Johns Hopkins University Population Communication Services (PCS). Ms. Leibtag has worked as a cataloguer/reference librarian at the JHU Population Dynamics/Maternal and Child Health Library and as an abstractor and indexer for PIP. She is particularly experienced in the cataloging and maintenance of special collections.

Ruth Lopez is a health education coordinator with Salud Para la Gente Clinic's *Proyecto Alarma SIDA,* an AIDS prevention education program in Watsonville, California. She brings to her work a unique perspective based on her life experience. Ms. Lopez is a bilingual, bicultural, biliterate Chicana/Native American. She has done extensive historical research on the relationship between Native Americans and Chicanos in the American Southwest. She worked for five years as a community organizer with the North Mission Association in San Francisco, California. She also has four years of experience in marketing and sales. In addition, she worked for two years with the State of California Department of Health Services in the area of sexually transmitted disease control.

Shelley Mann, MPH, is the resource center director at Education Programs Associates (EPA), a nonprofit education and training organization in Campbell, California. She has developed and evaluated numerous health education materials targeted at high-risk populations. She is currently developing a series of educational materials addressing the relationship between drug and alcohol use and HIV infection, and is the author of the Parent-Teen AIDS Education Project program manual and brochure published by the San Francisco AIDS Foundation. With other EPA staff, Ms. Mann has provided training and consultation to hundreds of health care professionals on the evaluation and development of health education materials.

Ana Consuelo Matiella, MA is editor and staff writer for ETR Associates/Network Publications in Santa Cruz, California. She is the series editor for ETR Associates' Latino Family Life Education Curriculum Series and has written two of the units in the series: *Cultural Pride* and *La Familia* (1988). She has authored two activity books for children, *The Multicultural Caterpillar* and *We Are a Family* (1990, ETR Associates). Additionally, Ms. Matiella is in charge of materials development for the California AIDS Clearinghouse. One of her particular interests and areas of expertise is fotonovela production.

Hugh M. Rigby, BA, PGCE, is media materials coordinator at the Johns Hopkins University Population Services (PCS). A specialist in media materials development, Mr. Rigby manages the Media/Materials center, an international clearinghouse for the collection, distribution and production of print and audiovisual materials designed to promote family health. Mr. Rigby came to PCS from the Eastern and Southern Africa Regional Office for UNICEF, where he was visual communications officer for five years. Previously he practiced as a graphic designer developing media materials and was also a teacher of visual arts. A British citizen, Mr. Rigby holds an honors degree in design and a post graduate certificate in education.

Jane H. Root, PhD, has spent a professional lifetime contributing to the field of adult education for literacy. She is the coauthor of the training materials used world-wide by Literacy Volunteers of America and has served as the national president of that organization. She is also one of the authors of *Teaching Parents with Low Literacy Skills* (Doak, Doak and Root; Lippincott, 1985) and has been active in working with health professionals who are trying to reach the low-literacy audience. She is now a retired college professor and lives in Portland, Maine, where she writes and edits materials for health and welfare agencies.

Terry Tafoya, PhD, is a Taos Pueblo/Warm Springs Indian, currently on leave from his faculty appointments as professor of psychology at Evergreen State College and as clinical faculty of the University of Washington Medical School's Interpersonal Psychotherapy Clinic. He also serves as summer faculty for the Kinsey Institute in the area of cross-cultural sexuality, and is on the board of directors of the People of Color Against AIDS Network, a Washington state coalition for minority concerns. He is on the National AIDS Faculty for the American Psychological Association, and was one of the

founders of the National Native American AIDS Prevention Center.

Marna Copeland Taylor, MPH, directs training programs
for Education Programs Associates (EPA), a nonprofit
education and training organization in Campbell,
California. She served as the director of educational
materials at EPA for four years where she supervised
the development and evaluation of many AIDS-related
materials. She codirected a major evaluation of AIDS
education and training in California's state prison system and developed a series of educational materials for
prison inmates and staff. With other EPA staff, Ms.
Taylor has provided training and consultation to hundreds of health care professionals on the evaluation and
development of health education materials.

Stephen B. Thomas, PhD, is an assistant professor of
community health in the Department of Health Education and Codirector of the Minority Health Research
Laboratory at the University of Maryland in College
Park. He is chair of the Advisory Council on Racial and
Ethnic Minority Health in the State of Maryland, and
executive secretary of the Alcohol and Drug Section in
the American Public Health Association. Dr. Thomas
has earned a bachelor of science degree in school health
education from The Ohio State University, a master of
science degree in community health from Illinois State
University, and completed his doctoral degree in community health from Southern Illinois University in Car-
bondale. He conducted his doctoral research on voting
behavior of the U.S. Senate on health legislation from
1973-1982. Dr. Thomas is currently principal investigator
on a major grant from the Robert Wood Johnson Foundation titled "SAMM: Stopping AIDS is My Mission, A
Community Coalition Model for AIDS Education and

Risk Reduction in the Black Community." The program is being implemented in a low-income public housing complex in metropolitan Washington, DC. He believes that health professionals have a responsibility to increase the amount of teaching, service and research focused on underserved, poorly served and never served populations within our society.

Sala Udin is the cofounder and executive director of the Multicultural Training Resource Center (MTRC), established in 1983. Mr. Udin has been in the field of substance abuse treatment and prevention for 23 years, 11 years of which have been as a trainer and consultant. MTRC has been on the cutting edge of culturally relevant materials development and program design since 1984 and has produced award-winning videos, brochures, posters, comic and coloring books and booklets.

Douglas A. Wirth, BSW, is a social worker and serves as director of five homeless shelters in Green Bay, Wisconsin, that provide a national model of transition. He is on the board of directors for Center Project, Inc., an AIDS service organization serving 17 counties in Northeastern Wisconsin. Mr. Wirth is also the primary AIDS educator for the Amerindian Center of Green Bay, and is active in the Great Lakes region in AIDS prevention and multicultural concerns.